High-Yield™
Neuroanatomy

FOURTH EDITION

High-Yield™
Neuroanatomy
FOURTH EDITION

James D. Fix, PhD
Professor Emeritus of Anatomy
Marshall University School of Medicine
Huntington, West Virginia

With Contributions by
Jennifer K. Brueckner, PhD
Associate Professor
Assistant Dean for Student Affairs
Department of Anatomy and Neurobiology
University of Kentucky College of Medicine
Lexington, Kentucky

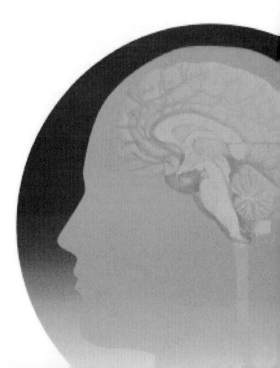

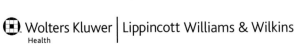
Wolters Kluwer | Lippincott Williams & Wilkins
Health
Philadelphia · Baltimore · New York · London
Buenos Aires · Hong Kong · Sydney · Tokyo

Acquisitions Editor: Crystal Taylor
Managing Editor: Kelley Squazzo
Marketing Manager: Emilie Moyer
Designer: Terry Mallon
Compositor: Aptara

Fourth Edition

351 West Camden Street   530 Walnut Street
Baltimore, MD 21201   Philadelphia, PA 19106

Printed in the United States of America.

9 8 7 6 5 4

Library of Congress Cataloging-in-Publication Data

Fix, James D.
    High yield neuroanatomy / James D. Fix, Jennifer K. Brueckner. — 4th ed.
        p. ; cm.
    Includes bibliographical references and index.
    ISBN 978-0-7817-7946-3
    1. Neuroanatomy—Outlines, syllabi, etc. 2.   Neuroanatomy—Examinations, questions, etc. I. Brueckner, Jennifer K., 1970- II. Title.
    [DNLM: 1.   Nervous System—anatomy & histology—Examination Questions. 2.   Nervous System—anatomy & histology—Outlines. 3.   Nervous System Diseases—Examination Questions. 4.   Nervous System Diseases—Outlines. WL 18.2 F566h 2009]
    QM451.F588 2009
    611'.8076—dc22

                                                                        2008024078

DISCLAIMER

Care has been taken to confirm the accuracy of the information present and to describe generally accepted practices. However, the authors, editors, and publisher are not responsible for errors or omissions or for any consequences from application of the information in this book and make no warranty, expressed or implied, with respect to the currency, completeness, or accuracy of the contents of the publication. Application of this information in a particular situation remains the professional responsibility of the practitioner; the clinical treatments described and recommended may not be considered absolute and universal recommendations.

The authors, editors, and publisher have exerted every effort to ensure that drug selection and dosage set forth in this text are in accordance with the current recommendations and practice at the time of publication. However, in view of ongoing research, changes in government regulations, and the constant flow of information relating to drug therapy and drug reactions, the reader is urged to check the package insert for each drug for any change in indications and dosage and for added warnings and precautions. This is particularly important when the recommended agent is a new or infrequently employed drug.

Some drugs and medical devices presented in this publication have Food and Drug Administration (FDA) clearance for limited use in restricted research settings. It is the responsibility of the health care provider to ascertain the FDA status of each drug or device planned for use in their clinical practice.

To purchase additional copies of this book, call our customer service department at (800) 638-3030 or fax orders to (301) 223-2320. International customers should call (301) 223-2300.

Visit Lippincott Williams & Wilkins on the Internet: http://www.lww.com. Lippincott Williams & Wilkins customer service representatives are available from 8:30 am to 6:00 pm EST.

Preface

Based on your feedback on previous editions of this text, the fourth edition has been reorganized and updated significantly. New features include chapter reorganization, terminology updates consistent with *Terminologica Anatomica*, addition of a table of common neurologic disease states, and an online ancillary of board-style review questions. To make the most effective use of this book, study the computed tomography scans and magnetic resonance images carefully and read the legends. Test your knowledge of each topic area with board-style questions provided online. Finally, remember these tips as you scan the chapters:

Chapter 1: What is the difference between Lewy and Hirano bodies? Nerve cells contain Nissl substance in their perikarya and dendrites but not in their axons. Remember that Nissl substance (rough endoplasmic reticulum) plays a role in protein synthesis. Study Figure 1-3 on the localization and prevalence of common brain and spinal cord tumors. Remember that in adults, glioblastoma multiforme is the most common brain tumor, followed by astrocytoma and meningioma. In children, astrocytoma is the most common brain tumor, followed by medulloblastoma and ependymoma. In the spinal cord, ependymoma is the most common tumor.

Chapter 2: The neural crest and its derivatives, the dual origin of the pituitary gland, and the difference between spina bifida and the Arnold-Chiari malformation are presented. Study the figures that illustrate the Arnold-Chiari and Dandy-Walker malformations.

Chapter 3: The mini-atlas provides you with the essential examination structures labeled on computed tomography scans and magnetic resonance images.

Chapter 4: Cerebrospinal fluid pathways are well demonstrated in Figure 4-1. Cerebrospinal fluid is produced by the choroid plexus and absorbed by the arachnoid villi that jut into the venous sinuses.

Chapter 5: The essential arteries and the functional areas that they irrigate are shown. Study the carotid and vertebral angiograms and the epidural and subdural hematomas in computed tomography scans and magnetic resonance images.

Chapter 6: The adult spinal cord terminates (conus terminalis) at the lower border of the first lumbar vertebra. The newborn's spinal cord extends to the third lumbar vertebra. In adults, the cauda equina extends from vertebral levels L-2 to Co.

Chapter 7: The important anatomy of the autonomic nervous system is clearly seen in Figures 7-1 and 7-2.

Chapter 8: The tracts of the spinal cord are reduced to four: corticospinal (pyramidal), dorsal columns, pain and temperature, and Horner's. Know them cold.

Chapter 9: Study the eight classic national board lesions of the spinal cord. Four heavy hitters are the Brown-Sequard syndrome, B_{12} avitaminosis (subacute combined degeneration), syringomyelia, and amyotrophic lateral sclerosis (Lou Gehrig's disease).

Chapter 10: Study the transverse sections of the brain stem and localize the cranial nerve nuclei. Study the ventral surface of the brain stem and identify the exiting and entering cranial nerves. On the dorsal surface of the brain stem, identify the only exiting cranial nerve, the trochlear nerve.

Chapter 11: This chapter on the cranial nerves is pivotal. It spawns more neuroanatomy examination questions than any other chapter. Carefully study all of the figures and legends. The seventh cranial nerve deserves special consideration (see Figures 11-5 and 11-6). Understand the difference between an upper motor neuron and a lower motor neuron (Bell's palsy).

Chapter 12: Cranial nerve (CN) V-1 is the afferent limb of the corneal reflex. CN V-1, V-2, III, IV, and VI and the postganglionic sympathetic fibers are all found in the cavernous sinus.

Chapter 13: Figure 13-1 shows the auditory pathway. What are the causes of conduction and sensorineural deafness? Describe the Weber and Rinne tuning fork tests. Remember that the auditory nerve and the organ of Corti are derived from the otic placode.

Chapter 14: This chapter describes the two types of vestibular nystagmus: postrotational and caloric (COWS acronym). Vestibuloocular reflexes in the unconscious patient are also discussed (see Figure 14-3).

Chapter 15: Know the lesions of the visual system. How are quadrantanopias created? There are two major lesions of the optic chiasm. Know them! What is Meyer's loop?

Chapter 16: The three most important lesions of the brain stem are occlusion of the anterior spinal artery (Figure 16-1), occlusion of the posterior inferior cerebellar artery (Figure 16-1), and medial longitudinal fasciculus syndrome (Figure 16-2). Weber's syndrome is the most common midbrain lesion (Figure 16-3).

Chapter 17: Figure 17-1 shows everything you need to know about what goes in and what comes out of the thalamus. Know the anatomy of the internal capsule; it will be on the examination. What is the blood supply of the internal capsule (stroke)?

Chapter 18: Figures 18-1 and 18-2 show that the paraventricular and supraoptic nuclei synthesize and release antidiuretic hormone and oxytocin. The suprachiasmatic nucleus receives direct input from the retina and plays a role in the regulation of circadian rhythms.

Chapter 19: Bilateral lesions of the amygdala result in Klüver-Bucy syndrome. Recall the triad hyperphagia, hypersexuality, and psychic blindness. Memory loss is associated with bilateral lesions of the hippocampus. Wernicke's encephalopathy results from a deficiency of thiamine (vitamin B_1). Lesions are found in the mamillary bodies, thalamus, and midbrain tegmentum (Figure 19-3). Know the Papez circuit, a common board question.

Chapter 20: Figure 20-1 shows the most important cerebellar circuit. The inhibitory γ-aminobutyric acid (GABA)-ergic Purkinje cells give rise to the cerebello-dentatothalamic tract. What are mossy and climbing fibers?

Chapter 21: Figure 21-6 shows the circuitry of the basal ganglia and their associated neurotransmitters. Parkinson's disease is associated with a depopulation of neurons in the substantia nigra. Huntington's disease results in a loss of nerve cells in the caudate nucleus and putamen. Hemiballism results from infarction of the contralateral subthalamic nucleus.

Chapter 22: This chapter describes the cortical localization of functional areas of the brain. How does the dominant hemisphere differ from the nondominant hemisphere? Figure 22-5 shows the effects of various major hemispheric lesions. What symptoms result from a lesion of the right inferior parietal lobe? What is Gerstmann's syndrome?

Chapter 23: In this chapter, the pathways of the major neurotransmitters are shown in separate brain maps. Glutamate is the major excitatory transmitter of the brain; GABA is the major inhibitory transmitter. Purkinje cells of the cerebellum are GABA-ergic. In Alzheimer's disease, there is a loss of acetylcholinergic neurons in the basal nucleus of Meynert. In Parkinson's disease, there is a loss of dopaminergic neurons in the substantia nigra.

Chapter 24: This chapter describes apraxia, aphasia, and dysprosody. Be able to differentiate Broca's aphasia from Wernicke's aphasia. What is conduction aphasia? This is board-relevant material.

While we have worked hard to ensure accuracy, we appreciate that some errors and omissions may have escaped our attention. We would welcome your comments and suggestions to improve this book in subsequent editions.

We wish you good luck.

James D. Fix
Jennifer K. Brueckner

Acknowledgments

The authors applaud all of the individuals at Lippincott Williams & Wilkins involved in this revision, including Crystal Taylor, Kelley Squazzo, Jennifer Verbiar, and Wendy Druck, Aptara Project Manager. Without their hard work, dedication, cooperation, and understanding, our vision for this new edition would not have been realized.

Acknowledgments

Contents

High-Yield™

Neuroanatomy

FOURTH EDITION

Chapter 1

Neurohistology

 Key Concepts

1) What is the difference between Lewy and Hirano bodies?
2) Nerve cells contain Nissl substance in their perikarya and dendrites but not in their axons. Remember that Nissl substance (rough endoplasmic reticulum) plays a role in protein synthesis.
3) Study Figures 1-3 and 1-4 on the localization and prevalence of common brain and spinal cord tumors. Remember that, in adults, glioblastoma multiforme is the most common brain tumor, followed by astrocytoma and meningioma. In children, astrocytoma is the most common brain tumor, followed by medulloblastoma and ependymoma. In the spinal cord, ependymoma is the most common tumor.

I NEURONS are classified by the number of processes (Figure 1-1).

A. PSEUDOUNIPOLAR NEURONS are located in the spinal (dorsal root) ganglia and sensory ganglia of cranial nerves (CN) V, VII, IX, and X.

B. BIPOLAR NEURONS are found in the cochlear and vestibular ganglia of CN VIII, in the olfactory nerve (CN I), and in the retina.

C. MULTIPOLAR NEURONS are the largest population of nerve cells in the nervous system. This group includes motor neurons, neurons of the autonomic nervous system, interneurons, pyramidal cells of the cerebral cortex, and Purkinje cells of the cerebellar cortex.

D. There are approximately 10^{11} neurons in the brain and approximately 10^{10} neurons in the neocortex.

II NISSL SUBSTANCE is characteristic of neurons. It consists of rosettes of polysomes and rough endoplasmic reticulum; therefore, it has a role in protein synthesis. Nissl substance is found in the **nerve cell body (perikaryon)** and **dendrites**, not in the axon hillock or axon.

III AXONAL TRANSPORT mediates the intracellular distribution of secretory proteins, organelles, and cytoskeletal elements. It is inhibited by colchicine, which depolymerizes microtubules.

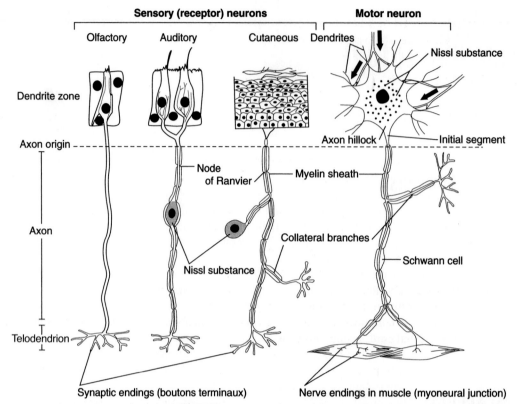

● **Figure 1-1** Types of nerve cells. Olfactory neurons are bipolar and unmyelinated. Auditory neurons are bipolar and myelinated. Spinal (dorsal root) ganglion cells (cutaneous) are pseudounipolar and myelinated. Motor neurons are multipolar and myelinated. *Arrows* indicate input through the axons of other neurons. Nerve cells are characterized by the presence of Nissl substance and rough endoplasmic reticulum. (Modified from Carpenter MB, Sutin J, *Human Neuroanatomy.* Baltimore: Williams & Wilkins, 1983:92, with permission.)

A. **FAST ANTEROGRADE AXONAL TRANSPORT** is responsible for transporting all newly synthesized membranous organelles (vesicles) and precursors of neurotransmitters. This process occurs at the rate of 200 to 400 mm/day. It is mediated by neurotubules and **kinesin**. (Fast transport is neurotubule-dependent.)

B. **SLOW ANTEROGRADE TRANSPORT** is responsible for transporting fibrillar cytoskeletal and protoplasmic elements. This process occurs at the rate of 1 to 5 mm/day.

C. **FAST RETROGRADE TRANSPORT** returns used materials from the axon terminal to the cell body for degradation and recycling at a rate of 100 to 200 mm/day. It transports **nerve growth factor, neurotropic viruses**, and toxins, such as **herpes simplex, rabies, poliovirus**, and **tetanus toxin**. It is mediated by neurotubules and **dynein**.

IV WALLERIAN DEGENERATION is anterograde degeneration characterized by the disappearance of axons and myelin sheaths and the secondary proliferation of Schwann cells. It occurs in the central nervous system (CNS) and the peripheral nervous system (PNS).

V **CHROMATOLYSIS** is the result of retrograde degeneration in the neurons of the CNS and PNS. There is a loss of Nissl substance after axotomy.

VI **REGENERATION OF NERVE CELLS**

A. **CNS.** Effective regeneration does not occur in the CNS. For example, there is no regeneration of the optic nerve, which is a tract of the diencephalon. There are no basement membranes or endoneural investments surrounding the axons of the CNS.

B. **PNS.** Regeneration does occur in the PNS. The proximal tip of a severed axon grows into the endoneural tube, which consists of Schwann cell basement membrane and endoneurium. The axon sprout grows at the rate of 3 mm/day (Figure 1-2).

VII **GLIAL CELLS** are the nonneural cells of the nervous system.

A. **MACROGLIA** consist of **astrocytes and oligodendrocytes**.
  1. **Astrocytes** perform the following functions:
    a. They project foot processes that envelop the basement membrane of capillaries, neurons, and synapses.
    b. They form the external and internal glial-limiting membranes of the CNS.
    c. They play a role in the metabolism of certain neurotransmitters [e.g., γ-aminobutyric acid (GABA), serotonin, glutamate].
    d. They buffer the potassium concentration of the extracellular space.
    e. They form glial scars in damaged areas of the brain (i.e., astrogliosis).
    f. They contain glial fibrillary acidic protein (GFAP), which is a marker for astrocytes.
    g. They contain glutamine synthetase, another biochemical marker for astrocytes.
    h. They may be identified with monoclonal antibodies (e.g., A_2B_5).
  2. **Oligodendrocytes** are the myelin-forming cells of the CNS. One oligodendrocyte can myelinate as many as 30 axons.

B. **MICROGLIA** arise from monocytes and function as the scavenger cells (phagocytes) of the CNS.

C. **EPENDYMAL CELLS** are ciliated cells that line the central canal and ventricles of the brain. They also line the luminal surface of the choroid plexus. These cells **produce cerebrospinal fluid (CSF)**.

D. **TANYCYTES** are modified ependymal cells that contact capillaries and neurons. They mediate cellular transport between the ventricles and the neuropil. They project to hypothalamic nuclei that regulate the release of gonadotropic hormone from the adenohypophysis.

E. **SCHWANN CELLS** are derived from the neural crest. They are the myelin-forming cells of the PNS. One Schwann cell can myelinate only one internode. Schwann cells invest all myelinated and unmyelinated axons of the PNS and are separated from each other by the **nodes of Ranvier**.

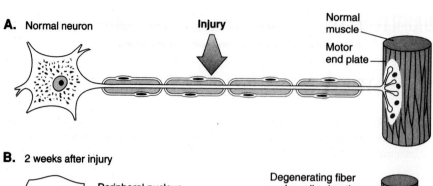

A. Normal neuron

Injury

Normal muscle

Motor end plate

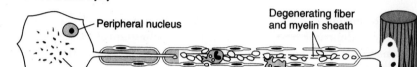

B. 2 weeks after injury

Peripheral nucleus

Degenerating fiber and myelin sheath

Fewer Nissl bodies

Macrophage

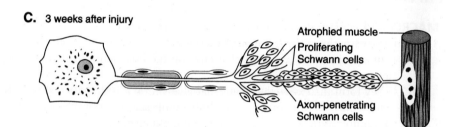

C. 3 weeks after injury

Atrophied muscle

Proliferating Schwann cells

Axon-penetrating Schwann cells

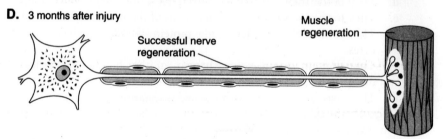

D. 3 months after injury

Muscle regeneration

Successful nerve regeneration

Unsuccessful nerve regeneration

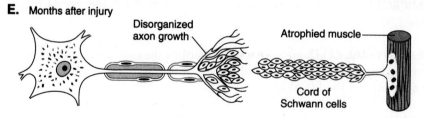

E. Months after injury

Disorganized axon growth

Atrophied muscle

Cord of Schwann cells

● **Figure 1-2** Schematic diagram of peripheral nerve regeneration.

VIII **THE BLOOD—BRAIN BARRIER** consists of the tight junctions of nonfenestrated endothelial cells; some authorities include the astrocytic foot processes. **Infarction of brain tissue** destroys the tight junctions of endothelial cells and results in **vasogenic edema**, which is an infiltrate of plasma into the extracellular space.

IX **THE BLOOD—CSF BARRIER** consists of the tight junctions between the cuboidal epithelial cells of the choroid plexus. The barrier is permeable to some circulating peptides (e.g., insulin) and plasma proteins (e.g., prealbumin).

X **PIGMENTS AND INCLUSIONS**

A. **LIPOFUSCIN GRANULES** are pigmented cytoplasmic inclusions that commonly accumulate with aging. They are considered residual bodies that are derived from lysosomes.

B. **MELANIN (NEUROMELANIN)** is blackish intracytoplasmic pigment found in the substantia nigra and locus coeruleus. It disappears from nigral neurons in patients who have Parkinson's disease.

C. **LEWY BODIES** are neuronal inclusions that are characteristic of Parkinson's disease.

D. **NEGRI BODIES** are intracytoplasmic inclusions that are pathognomonic of rabies. They are found in the pyramidal cells of the hippocampus and the Purkinje cells of the cerebellum.

E. **HIRANO BODIES** are intraneuronal, eosinophilic, rodlike inclusions that are found in the hippocampus of patients with Alzheimer's disease.

F. **NEUROFIBRILLARY TANGLES** consist of intracytoplasmic degenerated neurofilaments. They are seen in patients with Alzheimer's disease.

G. **COWDRY TYPE A INCLUSION BODIES** are intranuclear inclusions that are found in neurons and glia in herpes simplex encephalitis.

XI **THE CLASSIFICATION OF NERVE FIBERS** is shown in Table 1-1.

XII **TUMORS OF THE CNS AND PNS** are shown in Figures 1-3 and 1-4.

A. One-third of brain tumors are metastatic, and two-thirds are primary. In metastatic tumors, the primary site of malignancy is the lung in 35% of cases, the breast in 17%, the gastrointestinal tract in 6%, melanoma in 6%, and the kidney in 5%.

B. Brain tumors are classified as glial (50%) or nonglial (50%).

TABLE 1-1		CLASSIFICATION OF NERVE FIBERS	
Fiber	Diameter (μm)*	Conduction Velocity (m/sec)	Function
Sensory axons			
Ia (A-α)	12–20	70–120	Proprioception, muscle spindles
Ib (A-α)	12–20	70–120	Proprioception, Golgi tendon, organs
II (A-β)	5–12	30–70	Touch, pressure, and vibration
III (A-δ)	2–5	12–30	Touch, pressure, fast pain, and temperature
IV (C)	0.5–1	0.5–2	Slow pain and temperature, unmyelinated fibers
Motor axons			
Alpha (A-α)	12–20	15–120	Alpha motor neurons of ventral horn (innervate extrafusal muscle fibers)
Gamma (A-γ)	2–10	10–45	Gamma motor neurons of ventral horn (innervate intrafusal muscle fibers)
Preganglionic autonomic fibers (B)	<3	3–15	Myelinated preganglionic autonomic fibers
Postganglionic autonomic fibers (C)	1	2	Unmyelinated postganglionic autonomic fibers

*Myelin sheath included if present.

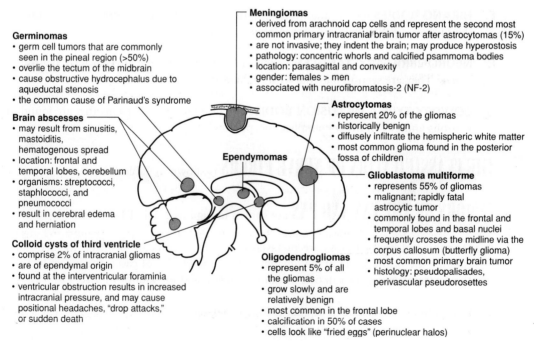

Meningiomas
- derived from arachnoid cap cells and represent the second most common primary intracranial brain tumor after astrocytomas (15%)
- are not invasive; they indent the brain; may produce hyperostosis
- pathology: concentric whorls and calcified psammoma bodies
- location: parasagittal and convexity
- gender: females > men
- associated with neurofibromatosis-2 (NF-2)

Germinomas
- germ cell tumors that are commonly seen in the pineal region (>50%)
- overlie the tectum of the midbrain
- cause obstructive hydrocephalus due to aqueductal stenosis
- the common cause of Parinaud's syndrome

Brain abscesses
- may result from sinusitis, mastoiditis, hematogenous spread
- location: frontal and temporal lobes, cerebellum
- organisms: streptococci, staphlococci, and pneumococci
- result in cerebral edema and herniation

Ependymomas

Astrocytomas
- represent 20% of the gliomas
- historically benign
- diffusely infiltrate the hemispheric white matter
- most common glioma found in the posterior fossa of children

Glioblastoma multiforme
- represents 55% of gliomas
- malignant; rapidly fatal astrocytic tumor
- commonly found in the frontal and temporal lobes and basal nuclei
- frequently crosses the midline via the corpus callosum (butterfly glioma)
- most common primary brain tumor
- histology: pseudopalisades, perivascular pseudorosettes

Colloid cysts of third ventricle
- comprise 2% of intracranial gliomas
- are of ependymal origin
- found at the interventricular foraminia
- ventricular obstruction results in increased intracranial pressure, and may cause positional headaches, "drop attacks," or sudden death

Oligodendrogliomas
- represent 5% of all the gliomas
- grow slowly and are relatively benign
- most common in the frontal lobe
- calcification in 50% of cases
- cells look like "fried eggs" (perinuclear halos)

● **Figure 1-3** Supratentorial tumors of the central and peripheral nervous systems. In adults, 70% of tumors are supratentorial. *CN*, cranial nerve; *CSF*, cerebrospinal fluid.

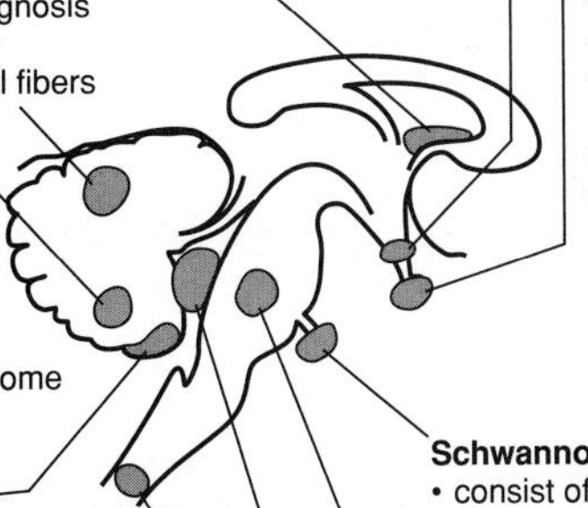

Choroid plexus papillomas
- historically benign
- represent 2% of the gliomas
- one of the most common brain tumors in patients < 2 years of age
- occur in decreasing frequency: fourth, lateral, and third ventricle
- CSF overproduction may cause hydrocephalus

Cerebellar astrocytomas
- benign tumors of childhood with good prognosis
- most common pediatric intracranial tumor
- contain pilocytic astrocytes and Rosenthal fibers

Medulloblastomas
- represent 7% of primary brain tumors
- represent a primitive neuroectodermal tumor (PNET)
- second most common posterior fossa tumor in children
- responsible for the posterior vermis syndrome
- can metastasize via the CSF tracts
- highly radiosensitive

Hemangioblastomas
- characterized by abundant capillary blood vessels and foamy cells; most often found in the cerebellum
- when found in the cerebellum and retina, may represent a part of the von Hippel-Lindau syndrome
- 2% of primary intracranial tumors; 10% of posterior fossa tumors

Intraspinal tumors
- Schwannomas 30%
- Meningiomas 25%
- Gliomas 20%
- Sarcomas 12%
- Ependymomas represent 60% of intramedullary gliomas

Craniopharyngiomas
- represent 3% of primary brain tumors
- derived from epithelial remnants of Rathke's pouch
- location: suprasellar and inferior to the optic chiasma
- cause bitemporal hemianopia and hypopituitarism
- calcification is common

Pituitary adenomas (PA)
- most common tumors of the pituitary gland
- prolactinoma is the most common (PA)
- derived from the stomodeum (Rathke's pouch)
- represent 8% of primary brain tumors
- may cause hypopituitarism, visual field defects (bitemporal hemianopia and cranial nerve palsies CNN III, IV, VI, V-1 and V-2, and postganglionic sympathetic fibers to the dilator muscle of the iris)

Schwannomas (acoustic neuromas)
- consist of Schwann cells and arise from the vestibular division of CN VIII
- compromise approx. 8% of intracranial neoplasms
- pathology: Antoni A and B tissue and Verocay bodies
- bilateral acoustic neuromas are diagnostic of NF-2

Brain stem glioma
- usually a benign pilocytic astrocytoma
- usually causes cranial nerve palsies
- may cause the "locked-in" syndrome

Ependymomas
- represent 5% of the gliomas
- histology: benign, ependymal tubules, perivascular pseudorosettes
- 40% are supratentorial; 60% are infratentorial (posterior fossa)
- most common spinal cord glioma (60%)
- third most common posterior fossa tumor in children and adolescents

● **Figure 1-4** Infratentorial (posterior fossa) and intraspinal tumors of the central and peripheral nervous systems. In children, 70% of tumors are infratentorial.

C. According to national board questions, the five most common brain tumors are
  1. **Glioblastoma multiforme,** the most common and most fatal type.
  2. **Meningioma,** a benign noninvasive tumor of the falx and the convexity of the hemisphere.
  3. **Schwannoma,** a benign peripheral tumor derived from Schwann cells.
  4. **Ependymoma,** which is found in the ventricles and accounts for 60% of spinal cord gliomas.
  5. **Medulloblastoma,** which is the second most common posterior fossa tumor seen in children and may metastasize through the CSF tracts.

XIII **CUTANEOUS RECEPTORS** (Figure 1-5) are divided into two large groups: free nerve endings and encapsulated endings.

A. Free nerve endings are nociceptors (pain) and thermoreceptors (cold and heat).

B. Encapsulated endings are touch receptors (Meissner's corpuscles) and pressure and vibration receptors (Pacinian corpuscles).

C. Merkel disks are unencapsulated light touch receptors.

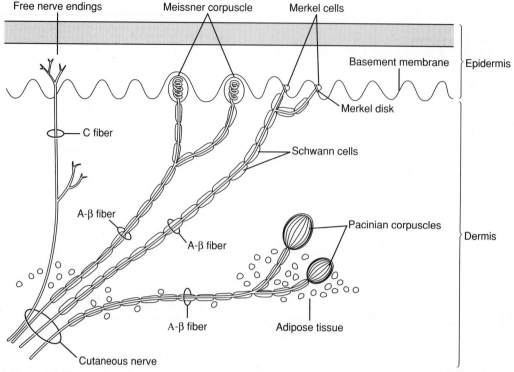

● **Figure 1-5** Three important cutaneous receptors. Free nerve endings mediate pain and temperature sensation. Meissner corpuscles of the dermal papillae mediate tactile two-point discrimination. Pacinian corpuscles of the dermis mediate touch, pressure, and vibration sensation. Merkel disks mediate light touch.

Case Study

A 44-year-old woman with a complaint of dizziness and ringing and progressive hearing loss in her right ear has a history of headaches. What is the most likely diagnosis?

Relevant Physical Exam Findings

• Unilateral sensorineural hearing loss

Relevant Lab Findings

• Radiologic findings show a right cerebellopontine angle mass that involves the pons and cerebellum.
• Neurologic workup shows discrimination impairment out of proportion to pure-tone thresholds.

Diagnosis

• Acoustic schwannomas are intracranial tumors that arise from the Schwann cells investing CN VIII (the vestibulocochlear nerve). They account for up to 90% of tumors found within the cerebellopontine angle. Cranial nerves V and VII are the next most common nerves of origin of schwannomas.

Chapter 2

Development of the Nervous System

Key Concepts

1) Be familiar with neural crest derivatives.
2) Recognizes the dual origin of the pituitary gland.
3) The difference between spina bifida and the Arnold-Chiari malformation.
4) Study the figures demonstrating Arnold-Chiari and Dandy-Walker malformations.

I THE NEURAL TUBE (Figure 2-1) gives rise to the **central nervous system (CNS)** (i.e., brain and spinal cord).

A. The **brain stem** and spinal cord have
   1. An **alar plate** that gives rise to the **sensory neurons.**
   2. A **basal plate** that gives rise to the **motor neurons** (Figure 2-2).

B. The neural tube gives rise to **three primary vesicles,** which develop into **five secondary vesicles** (Figure 2-3).

C. **ALPHA-FETOPROTEIN (AFP)** is found in the amniotic fluid and maternal serum. It is an indicator of neural tube defects (e.g., spina bifida, anencephaly). AFP levels are reduced in mothers of fetuses with Down syndrome.

II THE NEURAL CREST (see Figure 2-1) gives rise to

A. The **peripheral nervous system (PNS)** (i.e., peripheral nerves and sensory and autonomic ganglia).

B. The following cells:
   1. **Pseudounipolar ganglion cells of the spinal and cranial nerve** ganglia
   2. **Schwann cells** (which elaborate the myelin sheath)
   3. **Multipolar ganglion cells** of autonomic ganglia.
   4. **Leptomeninges** (the pia-arachnoid), which envelop the brain and spinal cord
   5. **Chromaffin cells** of the suprarenal medulla (which elaborate epinephrine).
   6. **Pigment cells** (melanocytes)
   7. **Odontoblasts** (which elaborate predentin)
   8. **Aorticopulmonary septum** of the heart
   9. **Parafollicular cells** (calcitonin-producing C-cells)
   10. **Skeletal** and **connective tissue components** of the **pharyngeal arches**

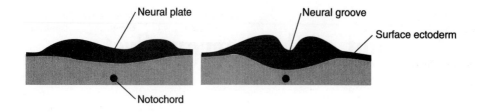

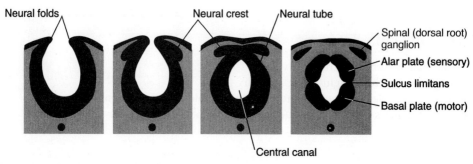

● **Figure 2-1** Development of the neural tube and crest. The alar plate gives rise to sensory neurons. The basal plate gives rise to motor neurons. The neural crest gives rise to the peripheral nervous system.

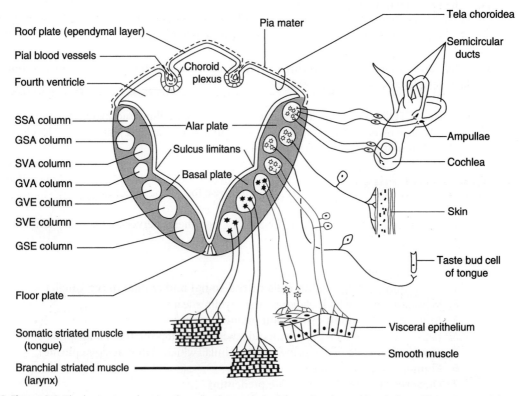

● **Figure 2-2** The brain stem showing the cell columns derived from the alar and basal plates. The seven cranial nerve modalities are shown. *GSA*, general somatic afferent; *GSE*, general somatic efferent; *GVA*, general visceral afferent; *GVE*, general visceral efferent; *SSA*, special somatic afferent; *SVA*, special visceral afferent; *SVE*, special visceral efferent. (Adapted from Patten BM. *Human Embryology,* 3rd ed. New York: McGraw-Hill, 1969:298, with permission.)

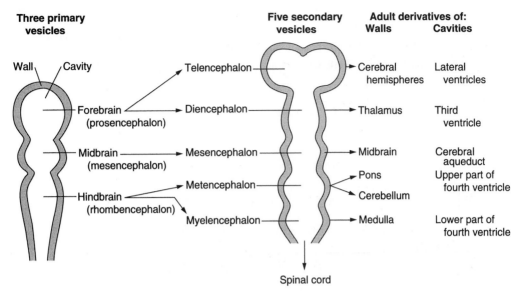

Three primary vesicles	Five secondary vesicles	Adult derivatives of: Walls	Cavities

Wall   Cavity

Telencephalon → Cerebral hemispheres / Lateral ventricles

Forebrain (prosencephalon) → Diencephalon → Thalamus / Third ventricle

Midbrain (mesencephalon) → Mesencephalon → Midbrain / Cerebral aqueduct

Metencephalon → Pons / Cerebellum / Upper part of fourth ventricle

Hindbrain (rhombencephalon) → Myelencephalon → Medulla / Lower part of fourth ventricle

Spinal cord

● **Figure 2-3** The brain vesicles indicating the adult derivatives of their walls and cavities. (Reprinted from Moore KL. *The Developing Human: Clinically Orienting Embryology,* 4th ed. Philadelphia: WB Saunders, 1988:380, with permission.)

III **THE ANTERIOR NEUROPORE** The closure of the anterior neuropore gives rise to the lamina terminalis. **Failure to close results in anencephaly** (i.e., failure of the brain to develop).

IV **THE POSTERIOR NEUROPORE** **Failure to close results in spina bifida** (Figure 2-4).

V **MICROGLIA** arise from the monocytes.

VI **MYELINATION** begins in the fourth month of gestation. Myelination of the corticospinal tracts is not completed until the end of the second postnatal year, when the tracts

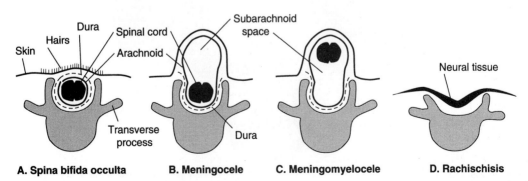

A. Spina bifida occulta   **B. Meningocele**   **C. Meningomyelocele**   **D. Rachischisis**

● **Figure 2-4** The various types of spina bifida. (Reprinted from Sadler TW. *Langman's Medical Embryology,* 6th ed. Baltimore: Williams & Wilkins, 1990:363, with permission.)

become functional. Myelination in the cerebral association cortex continues into the third decade.

A. **MYELINATION OF THE CNS** is accomplished by oligodendrocytes, which are not found in the retina.

B. **MYELINATION OF THE PNS** is accomplished by Schwann cells (Figure 2-5).

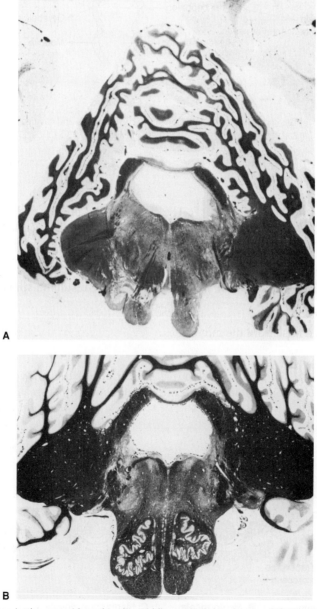

● **Figure 2-5** Myelination in the pyramids and in the middle cerebellar peduncles. **(A)** Nine months old; myelination incomplete. **(B)** Fifty-year-old adult; myelination is complete in all systems. (Reprinted from Haymaker W, Adams RD, *Histology and Histopathology of the Nervous System*. Springfield: Charles C Thomas, 1982:169, with permission.)

VII POSITIONAL CHANGES OF THE SPINAL CORD

A. In the **newborn**, the conus medullaris ends at the third lumbar vertebra (L-3).

B. In the **adult**, the conus medullaris ends at L-1.

VIII THE OPTIC NERVE AND CHIASMA are derived from the diencephalon. The optic nerve fibers occupy the **choroid fissure**. Failure of this fissure to close results in **coloboma iridis**.

IX THE HYPOPHYSIS (pituitary gland) is derived from two embryologic substrata (Figures 2-6 and 2-7).

A. **ADENOHYPOPHYSIS** (anterior lobe) is derived from an ectodermal diverticulum of the primitive mouth cavity (stomodeum), which is also called **Rathke's pouch**. Remnants of Rathke's pouch may give rise to a congenital cystic tumor, a **craniopharyngioma**.

B. **NEUROHYPOPHYSIS** (posterior lobe) develops from a ventral evagination of the hypothalamus (neuroectoderm of the neural tube).

X CONGENITAL MALFORMATIONS OF THE CNS

A. **ANENCEPHALY (MEROANENCEPHALY)** results from failure of the anterior neuropore to close. As a result, the brain does not develop. The frequency of this condition is 1:1,000.

B. **SPINA BIFIDA** results from failure of the posterior neuropore to form. The defect usually occurs in the sacrolumbar region. The frequency of spina bifida occulta is 10%.

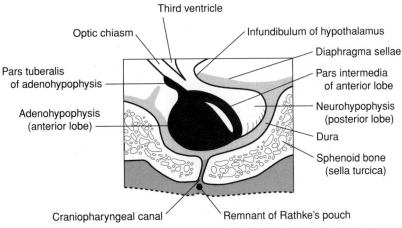

● **Figure 2-6** Midsagittal section through the hypophysis and sella turcica. The adenohypophysis, including the pars tuberalis and pars intermedia, is derived from Rathke's pouch (oroectoderm). The neurohypophysis arises from the infundibulum of the hypothalamus (neuroectoderm).

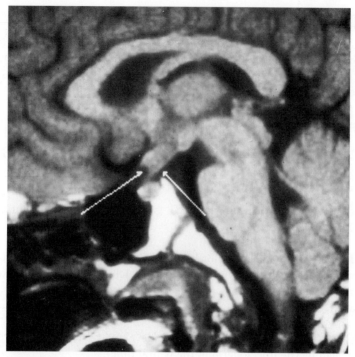

● **Figure 2-7** Midsagittal section through the brain stem and diencephalon. A craniopharyngioma (*arrows*) lies suprasellar in the midline. It compresses the optic chiasm and hypothalamus. This tumor is the most common supratentorial tumor that occurs in childhood and the most common cause of hypopituitarism in children. This is a T1-weighted magnetic resonance imaging scan.

C. **CRANIUM BIFIDUM** results from a defect in the occipital bone through which meninges, cerebellar tissue, and the fourth ventricle may herniate.

D. **ARNOLD-CHIARI** malformation (type 2) has a frequency of 1:1,000 (Figure 2-8). It results from elongation and herniation of cerebellar tonsils through foramen magnum, thereby blocking cerebrospinal fluid flow.

E. **DANDY-WALKER** malformation has a frequency of 1:25,000. It may result from riboflavin inhibitors, posterior fossa trauma, or viral infection (Figure 2-9).

F. **HYDROCEPHALUS** is most commonly caused by stenosis of the cerebral aqueduct during development. Excessive cerebrospinal fluid accumulates in the ventricles and subarachnoid space. This condition may result from maternal infection (cytomegalovirus and toxoplasmosis). The frequency is 1:1,000.

G. **FETAL ALCOHOL SYNDROME** is the most common cause of mental retardation. It includes microcephaly and congenital heart disease; holoprosencephaly is the most severe manifestation.

H. **HOLOPROSENCEPHALY** results from failure of midline cleavage of the embryonic forebrain. The telencephalon contains a singular ventricular cavity. Holoprosencephaly is seen in trisomy 13 (Patau syndrome); the corpus callosum may be absent. Holoprosencephaly is the most severe manifestation of the fetal alcohol syndrome.

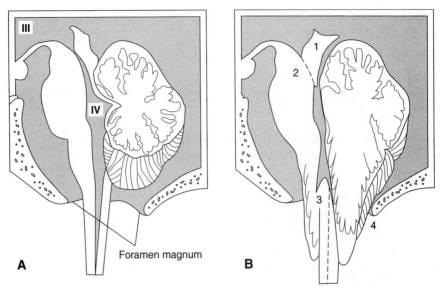

● **Figure 2-8** Arnold-Chiari malformation. Midsagittal section. **(A)** Normal cerebellum, fourth ventricle, and brain stem. **(B)** Abnormal cerebellum, fourth ventricle, and brain stem showing the common congenital anomalies: (*1*) beaking of the tectal plate, (*2*) aqueductal stenosis, (*3*) kinking and transforaminal herniation of the medulla into the vertebral canal, and (*4*) herniation and unrolling of the cerebellar vermis into the vertebral canal. An accompanying meningomyelocele is common. (Reprinted from Fix JD. *BRS Neuroanatomy*. Baltimore: Williams & Wilkins, 1996:72, with permission.)

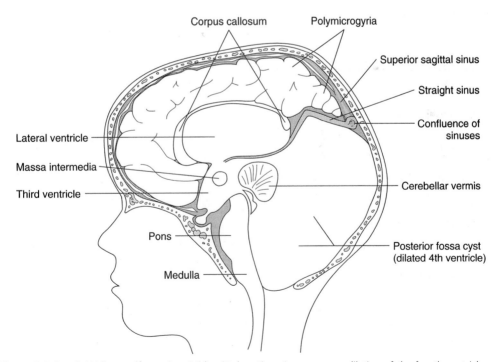

● **Figure 2-9** Dandy-Walker malformation. Midsagittal section. An enormous dilation of the fourth ventricle results from failure of the foramina of Luschka and Magendie to open. This condition is associated with occipital meningocele, elevation of the confluence of the sinuses (torcular Herophili), agenesis of the cerebellar vermis, and splenium of the corpus callosum. (Reprinted from Dudek RW, Fix JD. *BRS Embryology*. Baltimore: Williams & Wilkins, 1997:97, with permission.)

I. **HYDRANENCEPHALY** results from bilateral hemispheric infarction secondary to occlusion of the carotid arteries. The hemispheres are replaced by hugely dilated ventricles.

Case Study

A mother brings her newborn infant to the clinic because the infant's "legs don't seem to work right." The infant was delivered at home without antenatal care. What is the most likely diagnosis?

Relevant Physical Exam Findings

- Tufts of hair in the lumbosacral region
- Clubfoot (Talipes equinovarus)
- Chronic upper motor neuron signs, including spasticity, weakness, fatigability

Diagnosis

- Spina bifida occulta results from incomplete closure of the neural tube during week 4 of embryonic development. This type of neural tube defect often affects tissues overlying the spinal cord, including the vertebral column and skin.

Chapter **3**

Cross-Sectional Anatomy of the Brain

 Key Concepts

The mini-atlas provides you with the essential examination structures labeled on computed tomography scans and magnetic resonance images.

Ⅰ **INTRODUCTION** The illustrations in this chapter are accompanied by corresponding magnetic resonance imaging scans. Together they represent a **mini-atlas** of brain slices in the three orthogonal planes (i.e., midsagittal, coronal, and axial). An insert on each figure shows the level of the slice. The most commonly tested structures are labeled.

Ⅱ **MIDSAGITTAL SECTION** (Figures 3-1 through 3-3). The location of the structures shown in the figures should be known.

Ⅲ **CORONAL SECTION THROUGH THE OPTIC CHIASM** (Figures 3-4 and 3-5). The location of the structures shown in the figures should be known.

Ⅳ **CORONAL SECTION THROUGH THE MAMILLARY BODIES** (Figures 3-6 and 3-7). The location of the structures shown in the figures should be known.

Ⅴ **AXIAL IMAGE THROUGH THE THALAMUS AND INTERNAL CAPSULE** (Figures 3-8 and 3-9). The location of the structures shown in the figures should be known.

Ⅵ **AXIAL IMAGE THROUGH THE MIDBRAIN, MAMILLARY BODIES, AND OPTIC TRACT** (Figures 3-10 through 3-13). The location of the structures shown in the figures should be known.

Ⅶ **ATLAS OF THE BRAIN AND BRAIN STEM** (Figures 3-14 through 3-24). Included are midsagittal, parasagittal, coronal, and axial sections of thick, stained brain slices.

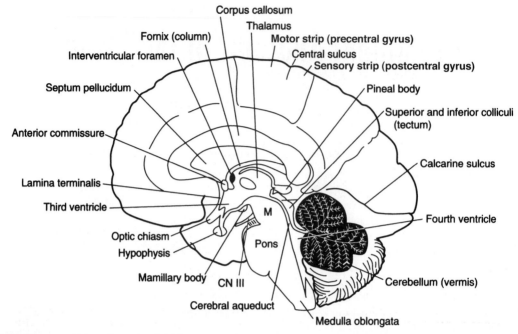

● **Figure 3-1** Midsagittal section of the brain and brain stem showing the structures surrounding the third and fourth ventricles. The brain stem includes the midbrain (*M*), pons, and medulla oblongata.

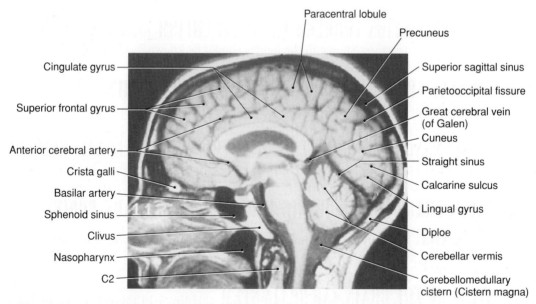

● **Figure 3-2** Midsagittal magnetic resonance imaging section through the brain and brain stem showing the important structures surrounding the third and fourth ventricles. This is a T1-weighted image. The gray matter appears gray (hypointense), whereas the white matter appears white (hyperintense).

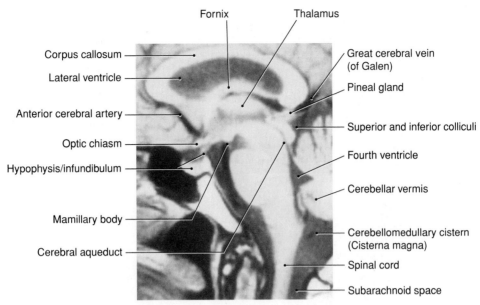

Fornix

Thalamus

Corpus callosum

Lateral ventricle

Anterior cerebral artery

Optic chiasm

Hypophysis/infundibulum

Mamillary body

Cerebral aqueduct

Great cerebral vein (of Galen)

Pineal gland

Superior and inferior colliculi

Fourth ventricle

Cerebellar vermis

Cerebellomedullary cistern (Cisterna magna)

Spinal cord

Subarachnoid space

● **Figure 3-3** Midsagittal magnetic resonance imaging section through the brain stem and diencephalon. Note the cerebrospinal fluid tract: lateral ventricle, cerebral aqueduct, fourth ventricle, cerebellomedullary cistern (cisterna magna), and spinal subarachnoid space. Note also the relation between the optic chiasm, infundibulum, and hypophysis (pituitary gland).

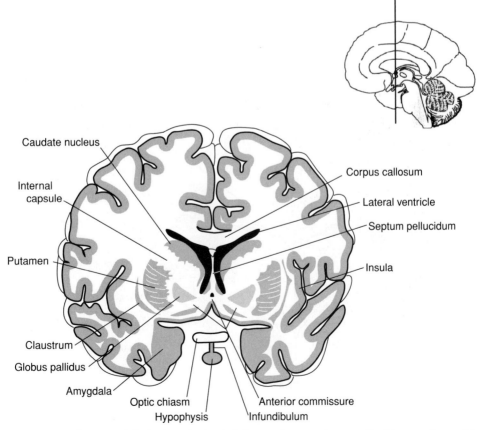

Caudate nucleus

Internal capsule

Putamen

Claustrum

Globus pallidus

Amygdala

Optic chiasm

Hypophysis

Corpus callosum

Lateral ventricle

Septum pellucidum

Insula

Anterior commissure

Infundibulum

● **Figure 3-4** Coronal section of the brain at the level of the anterior commissure, optic chiasm, and amygdala. Note that the internal capsule lies between the caudate nucleus and the lentiform nucleus (globus pallidus and putamen).

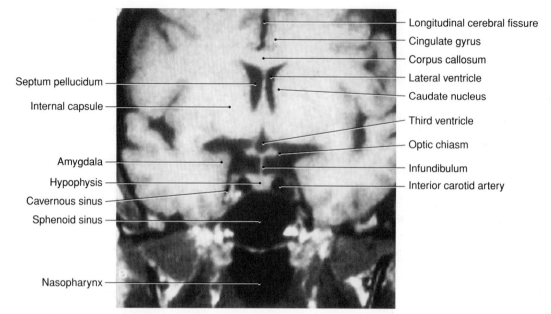

Septum pellucidum
Internal capsule

Amygdala
Hypophysis
Cavernous sinus
Sphenoid sinus

Nasopharynx

Longitudinal cerebral fissure
Cingulate gyrus
Corpus callosum
Lateral ventricle
Caudate nucleus
Third ventricle
Optic chiasm
Infundibulum
Interior carotid artery

● **Figure 3-5** Coronal magnetic resonance imaging section through the amygdala, optic chiasm, infundibulum, and internal capsule. The cavernous sinus encircles the sella turcica and contains the following structures: cranial nerves (CN) III, IV, VI, V_1, and V_2; postganglionic sympathetic fibers; and the internal carotid artery. This is a T1-weighted image.

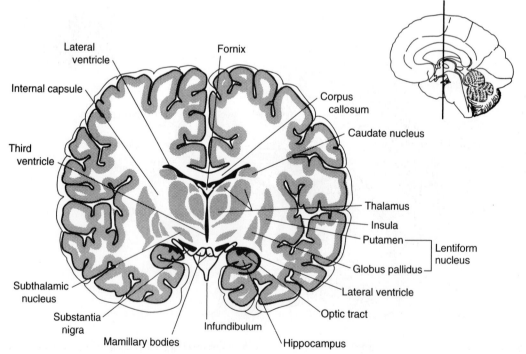

Lateral ventricle
Internal capsule
Third ventricle
Subthalamic nucleus
Substantia nigra
Mamillary bodies

Fornix
Corpus callosum
Caudate nucleus
Thalamus
Insula
Putamen
Lentiform nucleus
Globus pallidus
Lateral ventricle
Optic tract
Infundibulum
Hippocampus

● **Figure 3-6** Coronal section of the brain at the level of the thalamus, mamillary bodies, and hippocampal formation. Note that the internal capsule lies between the thalamus and the lentiform nucleus.

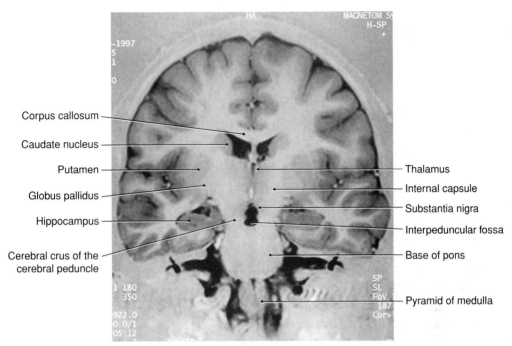

● **Figure 3-7** Coronal magnetic resonance imaging section of the brain and brain stem at the level of the thalamus, and hippocampal formation. Note that the posterior limb of the internal capsule lies between the thalamus and the lentiform nucleus (putamen and globus pallidus). This is a T1-weighted postcontrast image.

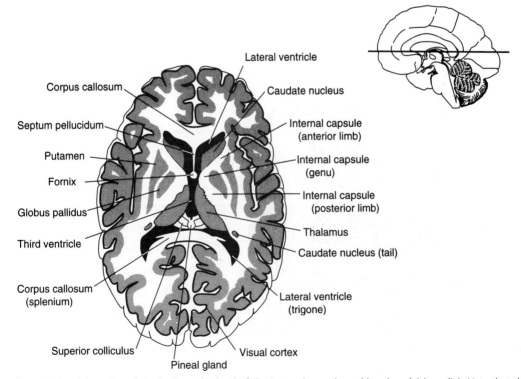

● **Figure 3-8** Axial section of the brain at the level of the internal capsule and basal nuclei (ganglia). Note that the internal capsule has an anterior limb, a genu, and a posterior limb. Note also that the corpus callosum is sectioned through the genu and splenium.

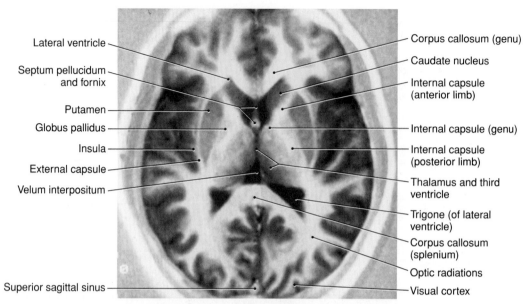

Lateral ventricle

Septum pellucidum and fornix

Putamen

Globus pallidus

Insula

External capsule

Velum interpositum

Superior sagittal sinus

Corpus callosum (genu)

Caudate nucleus

Internal capsule (anterior limb)

Internal capsule (genu)

Internal capsule (posterior limb)

Thalamus and third ventricle

Trigone (of lateral ventricle)

Corpus callosum (splenium)

Optic radiations

Visual cortex

● **Figure 3-9** Axial magnetic resonance imaging section at the level of the internal capsule and basal nuclei (ganglia). Note that the caudate nucleus bulges into the frontal horn of the lateral ventricle. In Huntington's disease, there is a massive loss of γ-aminobutyric acid (GABA)-ergic neurons in the caudate nucleus that results in hydrocephalus ex vacuo. A lesion of the genu of the internal capsule results in a contralateral weak lower face with sparing of the upper face. This is a T1-weighted image.

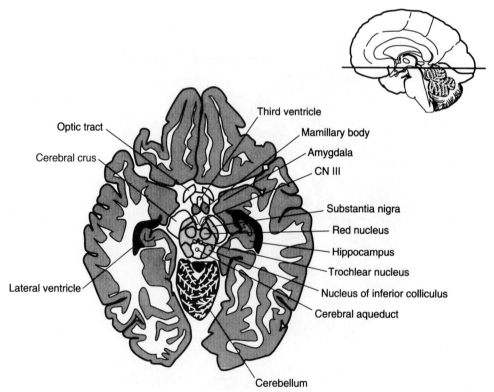

Optic tract

Cerebral crus

Lateral ventricle

Third ventricle

Mamillary body

Amygdala

CN III

Substantia nigra

Red nucleus

Hippocampus

Trochlear nucleus

Nucleus of inferior colliculus

Cerebral aqueduct

Cerebellum

● **Figure 3-10** Axial section of the brain at the level of the midbrain, mamillary bodies. Note that the substantia nigra separates the cerebral crus from the tegmentum of the midbrain.

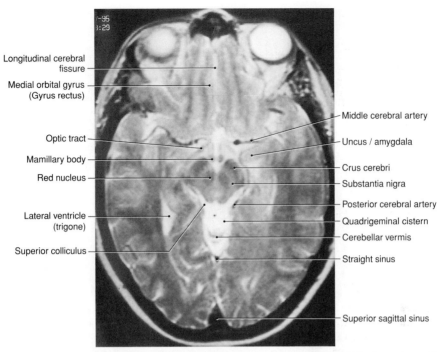

Longitudinal cerebral fissure
Medial orbital gyrus (Gyrus rectus)
Optic tract
Mamillary body
Red nucleus
Lateral ventricle (trigone)
Superior colliculus

Middle cerebral artery
Uncus / amygdala
Crus cerebri
Substantia nigra
Posterior cerebral artery
Quadrigeminal cistern
Cerebellar vermis
Straight sinus

Superior sagittal sinus

● **Figure 3-11** Axial magnetic resonance imaging (MRI) section at the level of the midbrain and mamillary bodies. Because of the high iron content, the red nuclei, mamillary bodies, and substantia nigra show a reduced MRI signal in T2-weighted images. Flowing blood in the cerebral vessels stands out as a signal void. Cerebrospinal fluid produces a strong signal in the ventricles and cisterns.

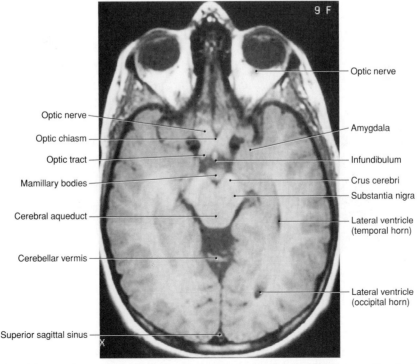

Optic nerve
Optic chiasm
Optic tract
Mamillary bodies
Cerebral aqueduct
Cerebellar vermis
Superior sagittal sinus

Optic nerve
Amygdala
Infundibulum
Crus cerebri
Substantia nigra
Lateral ventricle (temporal horn)
Lateral ventricle (occipital horn)

● **Figure 3-12** Axial magnetic resonance imaging section at the level of the optic chiasm, mamillary bodies, and midbrain. This patient has neurofibromatosis type 1 and an optic nerve glioma. Note the size of the right optic nerve. The infundibulum is postfixed. This is a T1-weighted image.

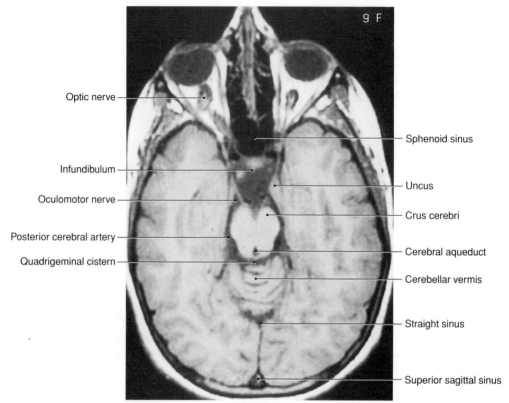

Optic nerve

Infundibulum

Oculomotor nerve

Posterior cerebral artery

Quadrigeminal cistern

Sphenoid sinus

Uncus

Crus cerebri

Cerebral aqueduct

Cerebellar vermis

Straight sinus

Superior sagittal sinus

● **Figure 3-13** Axial magnetic resonance imaging section at the level of the uncal incisure, oculomotor nerve. Is there pathology within the orbit?

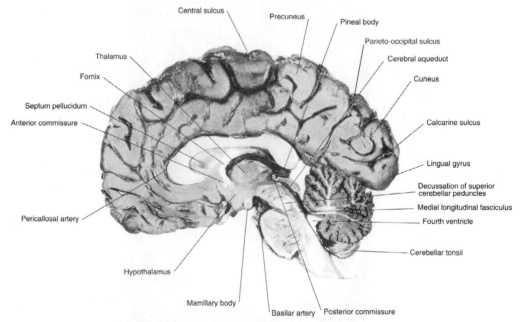

Central sulcus

Precuneus

Pineal body

Parieto-occipital sulcus

Thalamus

Cerebral aqueduct

Fornix

Cuneus

Septum pellucidum

Anterior commissure

Calcarine sulcus

Lingual gyrus

Decussation of superior cerebellar peduncles

Medial longitudinal fasciculus

Fourth ventricle

Pericallosal artery

Cerebellar tonsil

Hypothalamus

Mamillary body

Basilar artery

Posterior commissure

● **Figure 3-14** Gross midsagittal section of the brain and brain stem with meninges and blood vessels intact. Arachnoid granulations are seen along the crest of the hemisphere. The posterior commissure, decussation of the superior cerebellar peduncles, and medial longitudinal fasciculus are well demonstrated. (Reprinted from Roberts M, J Hanaway, DK Morest, *Atlas of the human brain in section,* 2nd ed. Philadelphia: Lea & Febiger, 1987:85, with permission.)

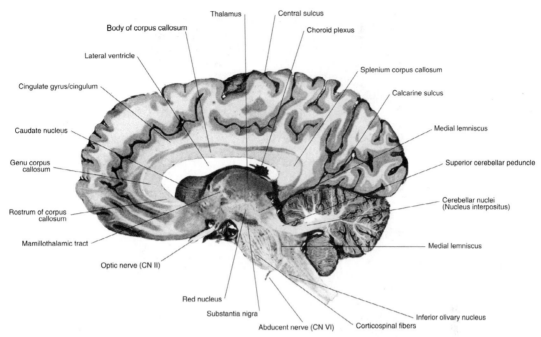

● **Figure 3-15** Gross parasagittal section through the red nucleus, medial lemniscus, and inferior olivary nucleus. The corticospinal fibers can be traced from the crus cerebri to the spinal cord. The abducent nerve (CN VI) is seen exiting from the pontonuclear sulcus. (Reprinted from M Roberts, J Hanaway, DK Morest, *Atlas of the human brain in section,* 2nd ed. Philadelphia: Lea & Febiger, 1987:81, with permission.)

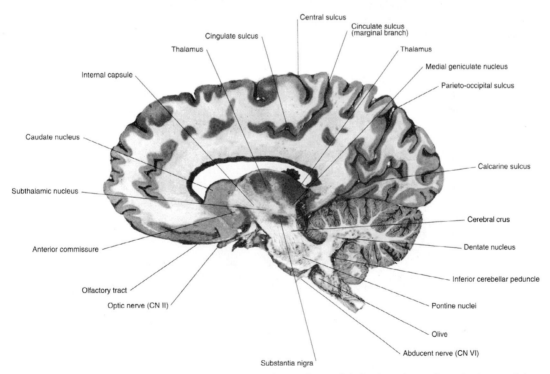

● **Figure 3-16** Gross parasagittal section through the caudate nucleus, subthalamic nucleus, substantia nigra, and dentate nucleus. The abducent nerve (CN VI) is seen exiting the pontobulbar sulcus. Damage to the subthalamic nucleus results in hemiballism. Parkinson's disease results from a cell loss of the pigmented neurons in the substantia nigra. (Reprinted from M Roberts, J Hanaway, DK Morest, *Atlas of the human brain in section,* 2nd ed. Philadelphia: Lea & Febiger, 1987:79, with permission.)

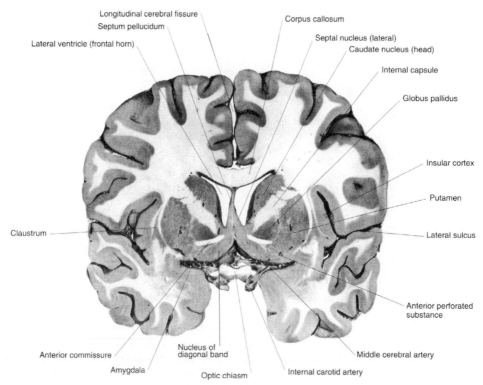

● **Figure 3-17** Coronal section through the anterior commissure, amygdala, septal nuclei, and optic chiasm. The septal nuclei have reciprocal connections with the hippocampal formation (subiculum). (Reprinted from M Roberts, J Hanaway, DK Morest, *Atlas of the human brain in section,* 2nd ed. Philadelphia: Lea & Febiger, 1987:9, with permission.)

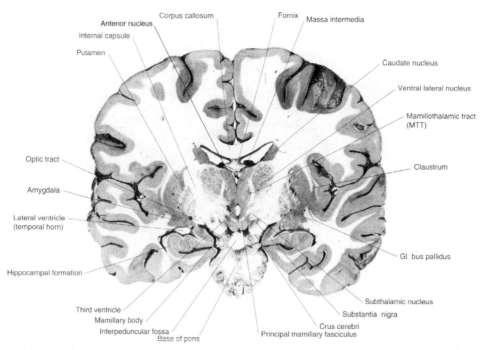

● **Figure 3-18** Coronal section through the posterior limb of the internal capsule, mamillothalamic tract (MTT), mamillary body, and hippocampal formation. Note the MTT entering the anterior ventral nucleus. The optic tracts are visible bilaterally. (Reprinted from M Roberts, J Hanaway, DK Morest, *Atlas of the human brain in section,* 2nd ed. Philadelphia: Lea & Febiger, 1987:19, with permission.)

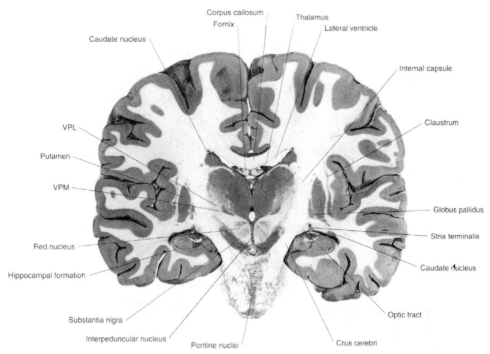

● **Figure 3-19** Coronal section through the thalamus, ventral posteromedial nucleus (*VPM*), and ventral posterolateral nucleus (*VPL*), posterior limb of the internal capsule, substantia nigra, and red nucleus. The optic tract lies dorsal to the temporal horn of the lateral ventricle. (Reprinted from M Roberts, J Hanaway, DK Morest, *Atlas of the human brain in section,* 2nd ed. Philadelphia: Lea & Febiger, 1987:23, with permission.)

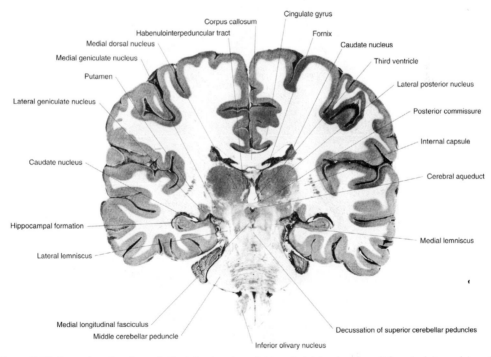

● **Figure 3-20** Coronal section through the lateral and medial lemnisci, lateral and medial geniculate nuclei, and hippocampal formation. (Reprinted from M Roberts, J Hanaway, DK Morest, *Atlas of the human brain in section,* 2nd ed. Philadelphia: Lea & Febiger, 1987:25, with permission.)

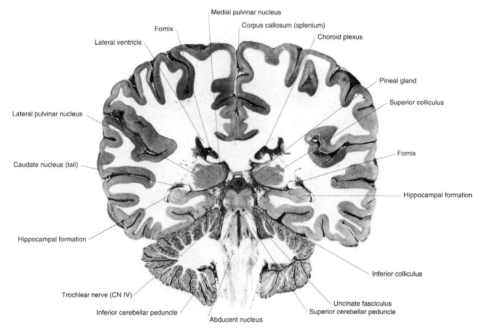

● **Figure 3-21** Coronal section through the pulvinar nuclei, pineal gland (epiphysis), superior and inferior colliculi, and trochlear nerve (CN IV). (Reprinted from M Roberts, J Hanaway, DK Morest, *Atlas of the human brain in section,* 2nd ed. Philadelphia: Lea & Febiger, 1987:29, with permission.)

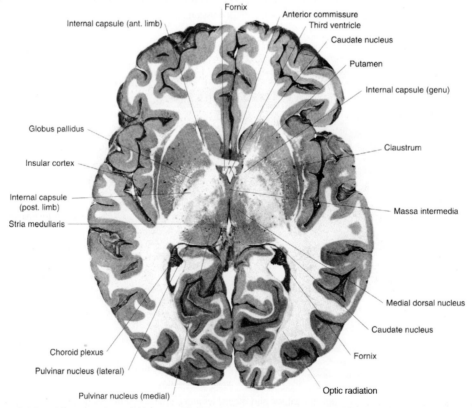

● **Figure 3-22** Axial section through the internal capsule, anterior commissure, and pulvinar nuclei. (Reprinted from M Roberts, J Hanaway, DK Morest, *Atlas of the human brain in section,* 2nd ed. Philadelphia: Lea & Febiger, 1987:51, with permission.)

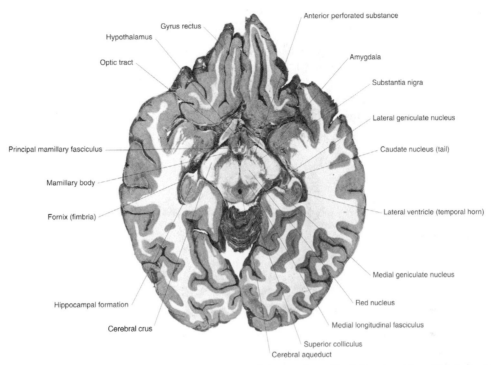

● **Figure 3-23** Axial section through the mamillary nuclei and the superior colliculi. (Reprinted from M Roberts, J Hanaway, DK Morest, *Atlas of the human brain in section,* 2nd ed. Philadelphia: Lea & Febiger, 1987:57, with permission.)

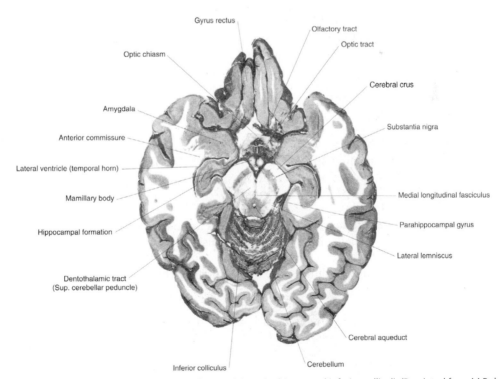

● **Figure 3-24** Axial section through the mamillary nuclei, optic chiasm, and inferior colliculi. (Reprinted from M Roberts, J Hanaway, DK Morest, *Atlas of the human brain in section,* 2nd ed. Philadelphia: Lea & Febiger, 1987:59, with permission.)

Chapter 4

Meninges, Ventricles, and Cerebrospinal Fluid

Key Concepts

Cerebrospinal fluid is produced by the choroid plexus and absorbed by the arachnoid villi that protrude into the venous sinuses. Cerebrospinal fluid pathways are well demonstrated in Figure 4-1.

 MENINGES are three **connective tissue membranes** that surround the spinal cord and brain.

A. The meninges consist of the **pia mater, arachnoid mater,** and **dura mater.**
   1. The **pia mater** is a delicate, highly vascular layer of connective tissue. It closely covers the surface of the brain and spinal cord.
   2. The **arachnoid mater** is a delicate, nonvascular connective tissue membrane. It is located between the dura mater and the pia mater.
   3. The **dura mater** is the outer layer of meninges. It consists of dense connective tissue that is divided into an outer periosteal (endosteal) layer and an inner meningeal layer. The meningeal layer forms dural folds. Dural venous sinuses are located between periosteal and meningeal layers of dura mater.

B. MENINGEAL SPACES
   1. The **subarachnoid space** (Figure 4-1) lies between the pia mater and the arachnoid. It terminates at the level of the second sacral vertebra. It contains the cerebrospinal fluid (CSF).
   2. Subdural space
      a. In the **cranium,** the subdural space is traversed by "bridging" veins.
      b. In the **spinal cord,** it is a clinically insignificant potential space.
   3. Epidural space
      a. The **cranial epidural space** is a potential space. It contains the meningeal arteries and veins.
      b. The **spinal epidural space** contains fatty areolar tissue, lymphatics, and venous plexuses. The epidural space may be injected with a local anesthetic to produce a paravertebral ("saddle") nerve block.

C. MENINGEAL TUMORS
   1. Meningiomas are benign, well-circumscribed, slow-growing tumors. They account for 15% of primary intracranial tumors and are more common in women than in men (3:2). Ninety percent of meningiomas are supratentorial.

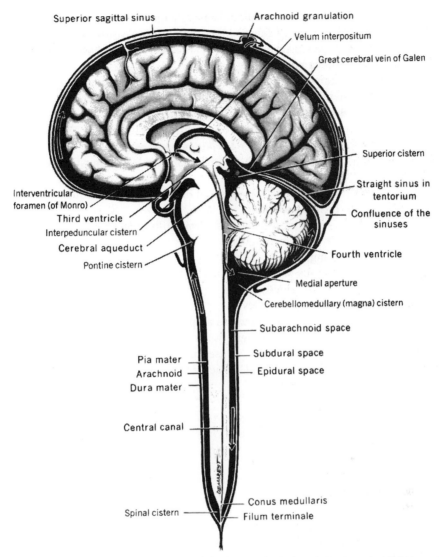

● **Figure 4-1** The subarachnoid spaces and cisterns of the brain and spinal cord. Cerebrospinal fluid is produced in the choroid plexuses of the ventricles. It exits the fourth ventricle, circulates in the subarachnoid space, and enters the superior sagittal sinus through the arachnoid granulations. Note that the conus medullaris terminates at L-1. The lumbar cistern ends at S-2. (Reprinted from CR Noback, NL Strominger, R Demarest, *The human nervous system,* 4th ed. Baltimore: Williams & Wilkins, 1991:68, with permission.)

2. **Subdural and epidural hematomas**
    a. **Subdural hematoma** is caused by laceration of the superior cerebral (bridging) veins.
    b. **Epidural hematoma** is caused by laceration of the middle meningeal artery.

E. **MENINGITIS** is inflammation of the pia–arachnoid area of the brain, the spinal cord, or both.
    1. **Bacterial meningitis** is characterized clinically by fever, headache, nuchal rigidity, and Kernig's sign. (With the patient supine, the examiner flexes the patient's hip but

cannot extend the knee without causing pain. It is a sign of meningeal irritation.) (Remember: Kernig = knee.) More than 70% of cases occur in children younger than 5 years. The disease may cause cranial nerve palsies and hydrocephalus.

   a. Common causes

      (1) In **newborns (younger than 1 month)**, bacterial meningitis is most frequently caused by *group B streptococci (Streptococcus agalactiae), Escherichia coli, and Listeria monocytogenes.*

      (2) In **older infants and young children (1 through 23 months)**, it is most commonly caused by *Streptococcus pneumoniae.*

      (3) In **young adults (2 through 18 years)**, it is most frequently caused by *Neisseria meningitidis.*

      (4) In **older adults (19 years and older)**, it is most frequently caused by *Streptococcus pneumoniae.*

      NB: Immunization against *Hemophilis influenzae* has significantly reduced this type of meningitis.

   b. CSF findings

      (1) Numerous polymorphonuclear leukocytes

      (2) Decreased glucose levels

      (3) Increased protein levels

2. Viral meningitis is also known as aseptic meningitis. It is characterized clinically by fever, headache, nuchal rigidity, and Kernig's sign.

   a. Common causes. Many viruses are associated with viral meningitis, including mumps, echovirus, Coxsackie virus, Epstein-Barr virus, and herpes simplex type 2.

   b. CSF findings

      (1) Numerous lymphocytes

      (2) Normal glucose levels

      (3) Moderately increased protein levels

Ⅱ VENTRICULAR SYSTEM

A. The **choroid plexus** is a specialized structure that projects into the lateral, third, and fourth ventricles of the brain. It consists of infoldings of blood vessels of the pia mater that are covered by modified ciliated ependymal cells. It secretes the CSF. Tight junctions of the choroid plexus cells form the blood–CSF barrier.

B. VENTRICLES CONTAIN CSF AND CHOROID PLEXUS

  1. The two **lateral ventricles** communicate with the third ventricle through the **interventricular foramina** (of Monro).

  2. The **third ventricle** is located between the medial walls of the diencephalon. It communicates with the fourth ventricle through the cerebral aqueduct.

  3. The **cerebral aqueduct** (of Sylvius) connects the third and fourth ventricles. It has no choroid plexus. Blockage of the cerebral aqueduct results in noncommunicating hydrocephalus.

  4. The **fourth ventricle** communicates with the subarachnoid space through three outlet foramina: two **lateral foramina** (of Luschka) and one **median foramen** (of Magendie).

C. HYDROCEPHALUS is dilation of the cerebral ventricles caused by blockage of the CSF pathways. It is characterized by excessive accumulation of CSF in the cerebral ventricles or subarachnoid space.

1. **Noncommunicating hydrocephalus** results from obstruction within the ventricles (e.g., congenital aqueductal stenosis).
2. **Communicating hydrocephalus** results from blockage within the subarachnoid space (e.g., adhesions after meningitis).
3. **Normal-pressure hydrocephalus** occurs when the CSF is not absorbed by the arachnoid villi. It may occur secondary to posttraumatic meningeal hemorrhage. Clinically, it is characterized by the triad of progressive dementia, ataxic gait, and urinary incontinence. (**Remember: wacky, wobbly, and wet.**)
4. **Hydrocephalus ex vacuo** results from a loss of cells in the caudate nucleus (e.g., Huntington's disease).
5. **Pseudotumor cerebri** (benign intracranial hypertension) results from increased resistance to CSF outflow at the arachnoid villi. It occurs in obese young women and is characterized by papilledema without mass, elevated CSF pressure, and deteriorating vision. The ventricles may be slitlike.

III **CEREBROSPINAL FLUID** is a colorless acellular fluid. It flows through the ventricles and into the subarachnoid space.

A. FUNCTION
1. **CSF supports the central nervous system (CNS) and protects it** against concussive injury.
2. It **transports hormones** and hormone-releasing factors.
3. It **removes metabolic waste products** through absorption.

B. FORMATION AND ABSORPTION. CSF is formed by the choroid plexus. Absorption is primarily through the arachnoid villi into the superior sagittal sinus.

C. The **composition of CSF** is clinically relevant (Table 4-1).
1. The normal number of **mononuclear cells** is fewer than $5/\mu L$.
2. **Red blood cells** in the CSF indicate subarachnoid hemorrhage (e.g., caused by trauma or a ruptured berry aneurysm).
3. **CSF glucose** levels are normally 50 to 75 mg/dL (66% of the blood glucose level). Glucose levels are normal in patients with viral meningitis and decreased in patients with bacterial meningitis.

TABLE 4-1	\multicolumn{4}{c}{CEREBROSPINAL FLUID PROFILES IN SUBARACHNOID HEMORRHAGE, BACTERIAL MENINGITIS, AND VIRAL ENCEPHALITIS}
Cerebrospinal Fluid	Normal	Subarachnoid Hemorrhage	Bacterial Meningitis	Viral Encephalitis
Color	Clear	Bloody	Cloudy	Clear, cloudy
Cell count/mm^3	<5 lymphocytes	Red blood cells present	>1,000 polymorphonuclear leukocytes	25–500 lymphocytes
Protein	<45 mg/dL	Normal to slightly elevated	Elevated, >100 mg/dL	Slightly elevated
Glucose ~66% of blood (80–120 mg/dL)	>45 mg/dL	Normal	Reduced	Normal

4. **Total protein levels** are normally between 15 and 45 mg/dL in the lumbar cistern. Protein levels are increased in patients with bacterial meningitis and normal or slightly increased in patients with viral meningitis.

5. **Normal CSF pressure** in the lateral recumbent position ranges from 80 to 180 mm H_2O. Brain tumors and meningitis elevate CSF pressure.

IV HERNIATION (Figures 4-2 through 4-7)

A. **TRANSTENTORIAL (UNCAL) HERNIATION** is protrusion of the brain through the tentorial incisure. This may result in oculomotor paresis and contralateral hemiplegia.

B. **TRANSFORAMINAL (TONSILLAR) HERNIATION** is protrusion of the brain stem and cerebellum through the foramen magnum. Clinical complications include obtundation and death.

C. **SUBFALCINE (CINGULATE) HERNIATION** is herniation below the falx cerebri. This condition does not necessarily result in severe clinical symptoms. It can present as headache. Compression of the anterior cerebral artery may result in contralateral leg weakness.

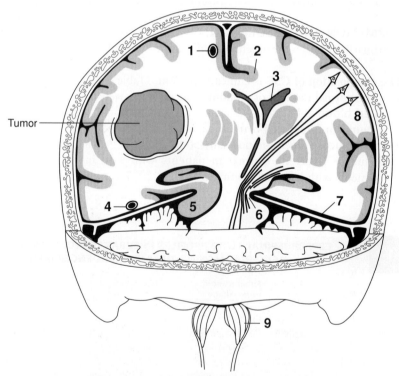

● **Figure 4-2** Coronal section of a tumor in the supratentorial compartment. (1) Anterior cerebral artery; (2) subfalcine herniation; (3) shifting of the lateral ventricles; (4) posterior cerebral artery (compression results in contralateral hemianopia); (5) uncal (transtentorial) herniation; (6) Kernohan's notch (contralateral cerebral peduncle), with damaged corticospinal and corticobulbar fibers; (7) tentorium cerebelli; (8) pyramidal cells that give rise to the corticospinal tract; (9) tonsillar (transforaminal) herniation, which damages vital medullary centers. (Adapted with permission from Leech RW, Shumann RM: *Neuropathology.* New York, Harper & Row, 1982, p. 16.)

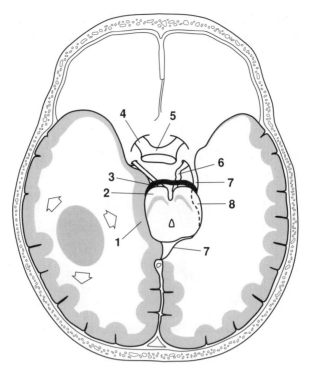

● **Figure 4-3** Axial section through the midbrain and the herniating parahippocampal gyrus. The left oculomotor nerve is being stretched (dilated pupil). The left posterior cerebral artery is compressed, resulting in a contralateral hemianopia. The right crus cerebri is damaged (Kernohan's notch) by the free edge of the tentorial incisure, resulting in a contralateral hemiparesis. Kernohan's notch results in a false localizing sign. The caudal displacement of the brain stem causes rupture of the paramedian arteries of the basilar artery. Hemorrhage into the midbrain and rostral pontine tegmentum is usually fatal (Duret's hemorrhages). The posterior cerebral arteries lie superior to the oculomotor nerves. *(1)* Parahippocampal gyrus; *(2)* crus cerebri; *(3)* posterior cerebral artery; *(4)* optic nerve; *(5)* optic chiasma; *(6)* oculomotor nerve; *(7)* free edge of tentorium; *(8)* Kernohan's notch. (Adapted from RW Leech, RM Shumann, *Neuropathology.* New York: Harper & Row, 1982:19, with permission.)

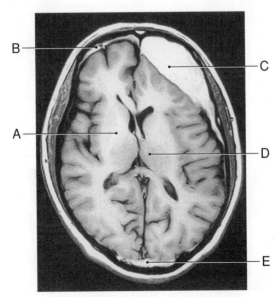

● **Figure 4-4** Magnetic resonance imaging scan showing brain trauma. *(A)* Internal capsule; *(B)* subdural hematoma; *(C)* subdural hematoma; *(D)* thalamus; *(E)* epidural hematoma. Epidural hematomas may cross dural attachments. Subdural hematomas do not cross dural attachments. The hyperintense signals are caused by methemoglobin. This is a T1-weighted image.

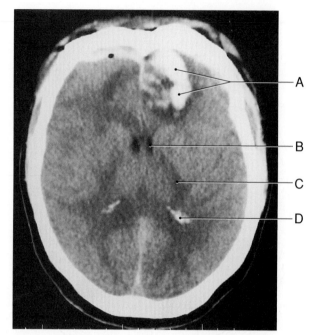

● **Figure 4-5** Computed tomography axial section showing an intraparenchymal hemorrhage in the left frontal lobe. (*A*) Intraparenchymal hemorrhage; (*B*) lateral ventricle; (*C*) internal capsule; (*D*) calcified glomus in the trigone region of the lateral ventricle.

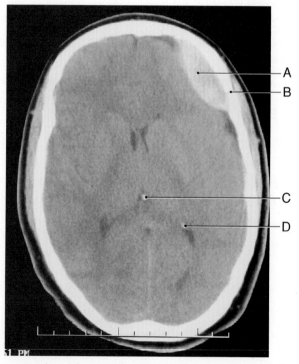

● **Figure 4-6** Computed tomography axial section showing an epidural hematoma and a skull fracture. (*A*) Epidural hematoma; (*B*) skull fracture; (*C*) calcified pineal gland; (*D*) calcified glomus in the trigone region of the lateral ventricle. The epidural hematoma is a classic biconvex, or lentiform, shape.

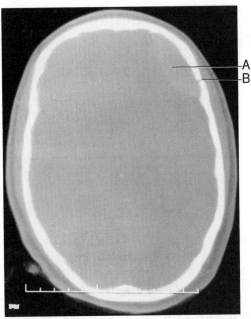

● **Figure 4-7** Computed tomography (CT) axial section showing a skull fracture (*A*) on the left side. An epidural hematoma (*B*) underlies the fracture. The CT scan shows a bone window.

 Case Study

The patient is a 68-year-old man with alcoholic cirrhosis. He fell 4 weeks ago. He has a history of progressive weakness on the right side. What is the most likely diagnosis?

Relevant Physical Exam Findings

- Hemiparesis
- Reflex asymmetry

Relevant Lab Findings

- Computed tomography scan of the head showed a crescent-shaped hypodense area between the cortex and skull. This mass has resulted in massive midline shift to the right, with subfalcine and uncal herniation.

Diagnosis

- Subdural hematoma results from bleeding between the dura mater and the arachnoid membrane from the bridging veins that connect the cerebral cortex to the dural venous sinuses. Subdural hematoma is common after acute deceleration injury from a fall or motor vehicle accident but rarely is associated with skull fracture.

Chapter 5

Blood Supply

 Key Concepts

1) The essential arteries supplying the brain and spinal cord and the functional areas that they irrigate
2) The carotid and vertebral angiograms and the epidural and subdural hematomas in computed tomography scans and magnetic resonance images

I **THE SPINAL CORD AND LOWER BRAIN STEM** are supplied with blood through the **anterior spinal artery** (Figure 5-1).

A. The anterior spinal artery supplies the **anterior two-thirds of the spinal cord**.

B. In the **medulla**, the anterior spinal artery supplies the pyramid, medial lemniscus, and root fibers of cranial nerve (CN) XII.

II **THE INTERNAL CAROTID SYSTEM** (see Figure 5-1) consists of the **internal carotid artery** and its branches.

A. The **ophthalmic artery** enters the orbit with the optic nerve (CN II). The **central artery of the retina** is a branch of the ophthalmic artery. Occlusion results in blindness.

B. The **posterior communicating artery** irrigates the hypothalamus and ventral thalamus. An **aneurysm** of this artery is the second most common aneurysm of the circle of Willis. It commonly results in **third-nerve palsy**.

C. The **anterior choroidal artery** arises from the internal carotid artery. It is not part of the circle of Willis. It perfuses the lateral geniculate body, globus pallidus, and posterior limb of the internal capsule.

D. The **anterior cerebral artery** (Figure 5-2) supplies the medial surface of the hemisphere from the frontal pole to the parietooccipital sulcus.
   1. The anterior cerebral artery **irrigates** the **paracentral lobule**, which contains the **leg-foot area of the motor and sensory cortices**.
   2. The **anterior communicating artery** connects the two anterior cerebral arteries. It is the most common site of **aneurysm** of the circle of Willis, which may cause **bitemporal lower quadrantanopia**.

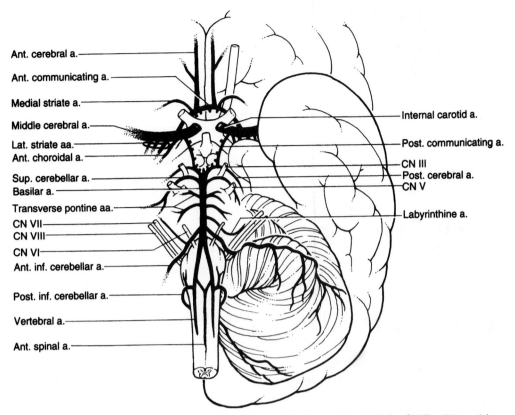

● **Figure 5-1** Arteries of the base of the brain and brain stem, including the arterial circle of Willis. *CN*, cranial nerve.

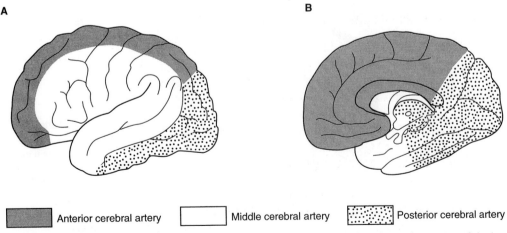

● **Figure 5-2** Cortical territories of the three cerebral arteries. **A:** Lateral aspect of the hemisphere. Most of the lateral convexity is supplied by the middle cerebral artery. **B:** Medial and inferior aspects of the hemisphere. The anterior cerebral artery supplies the medial surface of the hemisphere from the lamina terminalis to the cuneus. The posterior cerebral artery supplies the visual cortex and the posterior inferior surface of the temporal lobe. (Modified from Töndury, as presented in J Sobotta, *Atlas der anatomie des menschen*. Munich: Urban & Schwarzenberg, 1962:137–138.)

3. The **medial striate arteries** (see Figure 5-1) are the penetrating arteries of the anterior cerebral artery. They supply the anterior portion of the putamen and caudate nucleus and the anteroinferior part of the internal capsule.

E. The **middle cerebral artery** (see Figure 5-2)
    1. This middle cerebral artery supplies the lateral convexity of the hemisphere, including
        a. **Broca's and Wernicke's speech areas.**
        b. The **face** and **arm areas** of the motor and sensory cortices.
        c. The **frontal eye field.**
    2. The **lateral striate arteries** (Figure 5-3) are the penetrating branches of the middle cerebral artery. They are the arteries of **stroke**, and they supply the **internal capsule, caudate nucleus, putamen,** and **globus pallidus.**

Ⅲ THE VERTIBROBASILAR SYSTEM See Figure 5-1.

A. The **vertebral artery** is a branch of the subclavian artery. It gives rise to the **anterior spinal artery** (see I.) and the **posterior inferior cerebellar artery (PICA)**, which supplies the dorsolateral quadrant of the medulla. This quadrant includes the nucleus ambiguus (CN IX, X, and XI) and the inferior surface of the cerebellum.

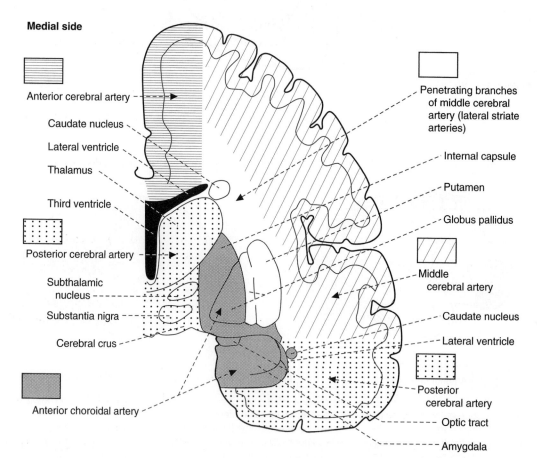

● **Figure 5-3** Coronal section through the cerebral hemisphere at the level of the internal capsule and thalamus, showing the major vascular territories.

B. The **basilar artery** is formed by the two vertebral arteries. It gives rise to the following arteries:

   1. The paramedian branches of the **pontine arteries** supply the base of the pons, which includes the corticospinal fibers and the exiting root fibers of the abducent nerve (CN VI).

   2. The **labyrinthine artery** arises from the basilar artery in 15% of people. It arises from the anterior inferior cerebellar artery in 85% of people.

   3. The **anterior inferior cerebellar artery (AICA)** supplies the caudal lateral pontine tegmentum, including CN VII, the spinal trigeminal tract of CN V, and the inferior surface of the cerebellum.

   4. The **superior cerebellar artery** supplies the dorsolateral tegmentum of the rostral pons (i.e., rostral to the motor nucleus of CN V), the superior cerebellar peduncle, the superior surface of the cerebellum and cerebellar nuclei, and the cochlear nuclei.

   5. The **posterior cerebral artery** (see Figures 5-1 through 5-3) is connected to the carotid artery through the posterior communicating artery. It provides the **major blood supply to the midbrain**. It also supplies the thalamus, lateral and medial geniculate bodies, and occipital lobe (which includes the visual cortex and the inferior surface of the temporal lobe, including the hippocampal formation). **Occlusion** of this artery results in a **contralateral hemianopia with macular sparing**.

IV **THE BLOOD SUPPLY OF THE INTERNAL CAPSULE** comes primarily from the **lateral striate arteries** of the middle cerebral artery and the **anterior choroidal artery**.

V **VEINS OF THE BRAIN**

A. The **superior cerebral ("bridging") veins** drain into the superior sagittal sinus. Laceration results in a **subdural hematoma**.

B. The **great cerebral vein** (of Galen) drains the deep cerebral veins into the **straight sinus**.

VI **VENOUS DURAL SINUSES**

A. The **superior sagittal sinus** receives blood from the bridging veins and **emissary veins** (a potential route for transmission of extracranial infection into brain). The superior sagittal sinus also receives cerebrospinal fluid (CSF) through the arachnoid villi.

B. The **cavernous sinus** contains CN III, IV, V-1 and V-2, and VI and the postganglionic sympathetic fibers. It also contains the siphon of the internal carotid artery (Figure 5-4).

VII **ANGIOGRAPHY**

A. **CAROTID ANGIOGRAPHY.** Figures 5-5A and B show the internal carotid artery, anterior cerebral artery, and middle cerebral artery.

B. **VERTEBRAL ANGIOGRAPHY.** Figures 5-5C and D show the vertebral artery, PICA and AICA, basilar artery, superior cerebellar artery, and posterior cerebral artery (Figures 5-6 and 5-7).

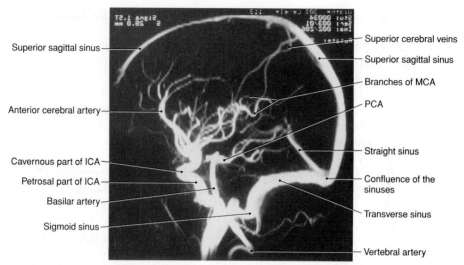

● **Figure 5-4** Magnetic resonance angiogram, lateral projection, showing the major venous sinuses and arteries. Note the bridging veins entering the superior sagittal sinus. *ICA,* internal carotid artery; *MCA,* middle cerebral artery; *PCA,* posterior cerebral artery.

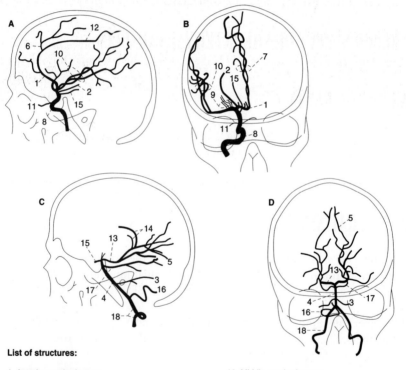

List of structures:

1. Anterior cerebral artery
2. Anterior choroidal artery
3. Anterior inferior cerebellar artery
4. Basilar artery
5. Calcarine artery (of posterior cerebral artery)
6. Callosomarginal artery (of anterior cerebral artery)
7. Callosomarginal and pericallosal arteries (of anterior cerebral artery)
8. Internal carotid artery
9. Lateral striate arteries (of middle cerebral artery)
10. Middle cerebral artery
11. Ophthalmic artery
12. Pericallosal artery (of anterior cerebral artery)
13. Posterior cerebral artery
14. Posterior choroidal arteries (of posteior cerebral artery)
15. Posterior communicating artery
16. Posterior inferior cerebellar artery
17. Superior cerebellar artery
18. Vertebral artery

● **Figure 5-5 A:** Carotid angiogram, lateral projection. **B:** Carotid angiogram, anteroposterior projection. **C:** Vertebral angiogram, lateral projection. **D:** Vertebral angiogram, anteroposterior projection.

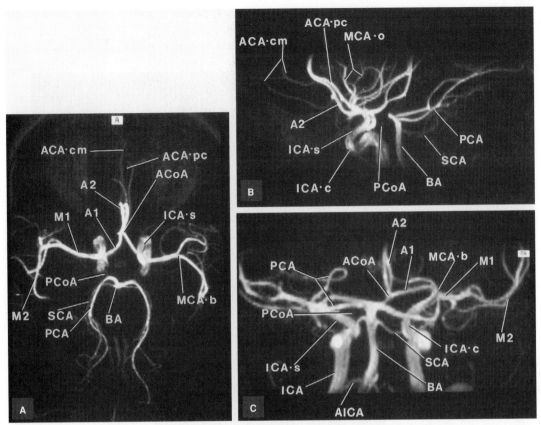

● **Figure 5-6** Arterial anatomy of a magnetic resonance section; axial **(A)**, sagittal **(B, C)**. *ACAcm*, anterior cerebral artery, callosal marginal branch; *A2* and *A1*, branches of the anterior cerebral artery; *ACApc*, pericallosal branch of the anterior cerebral artery; *ACoA*, anterior communicating artery; *AICA*, anterior inferior cerebellar artery; *M1* and *M2*, segments of the middle cerebral artery (*MCA*); *MCAb* = bifurcation; *ICAs*, internal carotid artery siphon; ICAc, internal carotoid artery cavernous *PCA*, posterior cerebral arterior, *PCoA*, posterior communicating artery; *BA*, basilar artery; *SCA*, superior cerebellar artery. (Reprinted from CB Grossman, *Magenetic resonance imaging and computed tomography of the head and spine*, 2nd ed. Philadelphia: Williams & Wilkins, 1996:124, with permission.)

C. **VEINS AND DURAL SINUSES.** Figure 5-8 shows the internal cerebral vein, superior cerebral veins, great cerebral vein, superior ophthalmic vein, and major dural sinuses.

D. **DIGITAL SUBTRACTION ANGIOGRAPHY.** See Figures 5-9 through 5-12.

VIII   **THE MIDDLE MENINGEAL ARTERY,** a branch of the **maxillary artery**, enters the cranium through the **foramen spinosum**. It supplies most of the dura, including its calvarial portion. Laceration results in **epidural hemorrhage** (hematoma) (Figures 5-13 and 5-14).

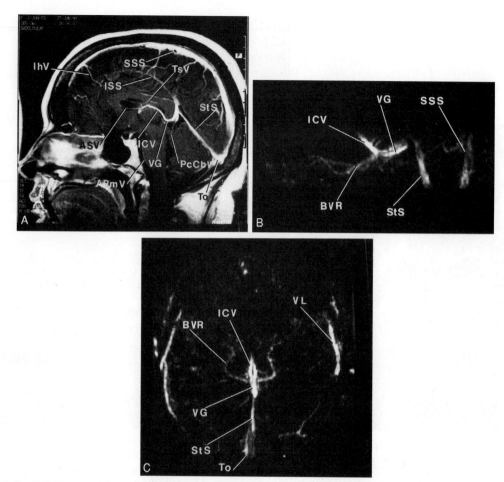

● **Figure 5-7** Venous anatomy of a magnetic resonance section; midsagittal **(A)**, lateral **(B)**, submental-vertex **(C)**. *IhV*, interhemispheric veins; *SSS*, superior sagittal sinus; *ISS*, inferior sagittal sinus; *TsV*, thalmostriate veins; *StS*, straight sinus; *PcCbV*, precentral cerebellar vein; *To*, torcula; *VG*, vein of anterior pontomesencephalic veins. (Reprinted from CB Grossman, *Magnetic resonance imaging and computed tomography of the head and spine*, 2nd ed. Philadelphia: Williams & Wilkins, 1996:125, with permission.)

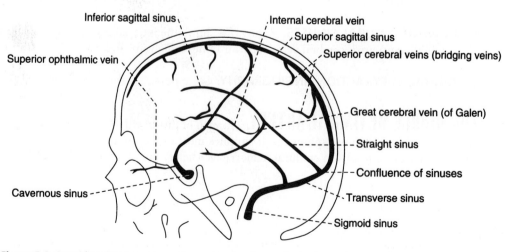

● **Figure 5-8** Carotid angiogram, venous phase, showing the cerebral veins and venous sinuses.

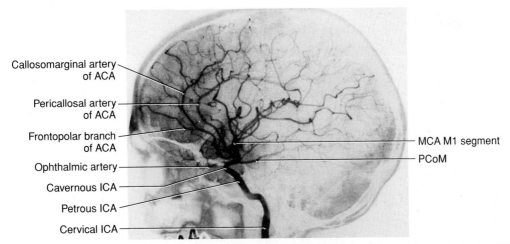

● Figure 5-9 Carotid angiogram, lateral projection. Identify the cortical branches of the anterior cerebral artery (*ACA*) and middle cerebral artery (*MCA*). Follow the course of the internal carotid artery (*ICA*). Remember that aneurysms of the posterior communicating artery (*PCoM*) may result in third-nerve palsy. The paracentral lobule is irrigated by the callosomarginal artery.

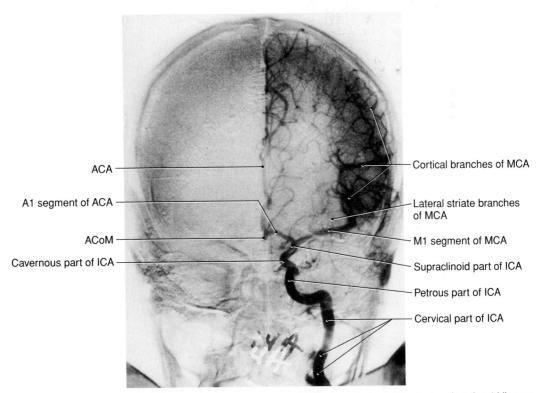

● Figure 5-10 Carotid angiogram, anteroposterior projection. Identify the anterior cerebral artery (*ACA*), middle cerebral artery (*MCA*), and internal carotid artery (*ICA*). The horizontal branches of the MCA perfuse the basal nuclei and internal capsule. *ACoM,* anterior communicating artery.

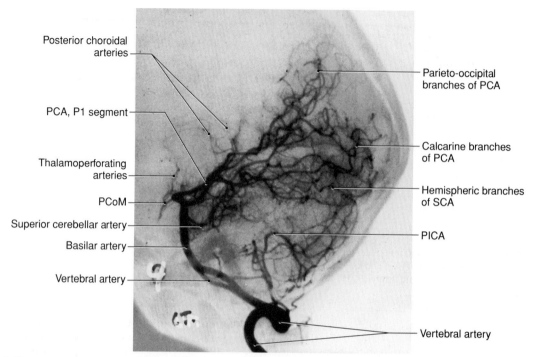

Posterior choroidal arteries

PCA, P1 segment

Thalamoperforating arteries

PCoM

Superior cerebellar artery

Basilar artery

Vertebral artery

Parieto-occipital branches of PCA

Calcarine branches of PCA

Hemispheric branches of SCA

PICA

Vertebral artery

● **Figure 5-11** Vertebral angiogram, lateral projection. Two structures are found between the posterior cerebral artery (*PCA*) and the superior cerebellar artery (*SCA*): the tentorium and the third cranial nerve. *PCoM,* posterior communicating artery; *PICA,* posterior inferior cerebellar artery.

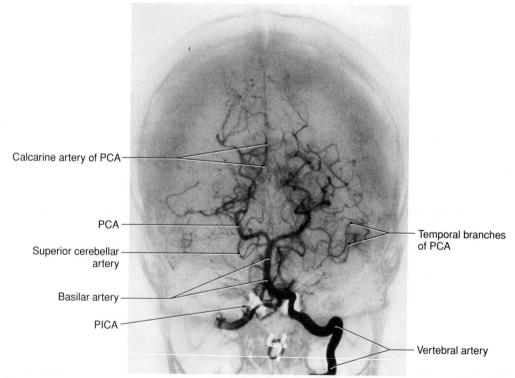

Calcarine artery of PCA

PCA

Superior cerebellar artery

Basilar artery

PICA

Temporal branches of PCA

Vertebral artery

● **Figure 5-12** Vertebral angiogram, anteroposterior projection. Which artery supplies the visual cortex? The calcarine artery, a branch of the posterior cerebral artery (*PCA*). Occlusion of the PCA (calcarine artery) results in a contralateral homonymous hemianopia, with macular sparing. *PICA,* posterior inferior cerebellar artery.

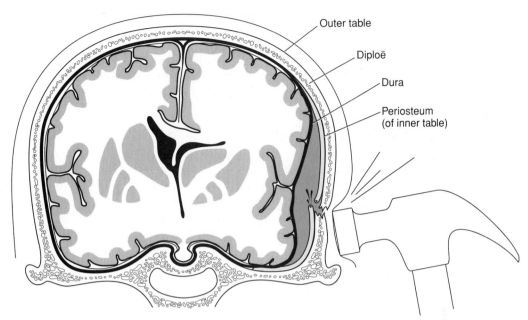

● Figure 5-13 An epidural hematoma results from laceration of the middle meningeal artery. Arterial bleeding into the epidural space forms a biconvex clot. The classic "lucid interval" is seen in 50% of cases. Skull fractures are usually found. Epidural hematomas rarely cross sutural lines. (Reprinted from AG Osburn, KA Tong, *Handbook of neuroradiology: brain and skull*. St. Louis: Mosby, 1996:191, with permission.)

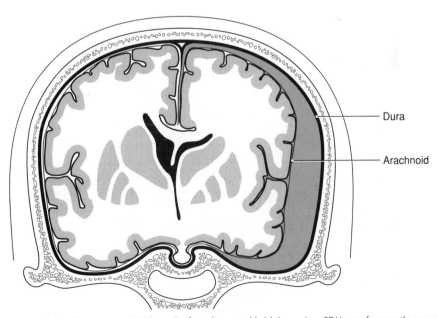

● Figure 5-14 A subdural hematoma (SDH) results from lacerated bridging veins. SDHs are frequently accompanied by traumatic subarachnoid hemorrhages and cortical contusions. Sudden deceleration of the head causes tearing of the superior cerebral veins. The SDH extends over the crest of the convexity into the interhemispheric fissure but does not cross the dural attachment of the falx cerebri. The clot can be crescent-shaped, biconvex, or multiloculated. SDHs are more common than epidural hematomas and always cause brain damage. (Reprinted from AG Osburn, KA Tong, *Handbook of neuroradiology: brain and skull*. St. Louis: Mosby, 1996:192, with permission.)

Case Study

A 62-year-old man comes to the clinic complaining of problems with his vision and a horrible headache that began earlier in the day. He reports bumping into objects and not being able to read half the printed page of the newspaper. He has a history of hypertension and diabetes mellitus. What is the most likely diagnosis?

Relevant Physical Exam Findings

- Complete hemianopia
- Contralateral face and limb sensory loss

Relevant Lab Findings

- Computed tomography scan of the brain determined the presence of ischemic infarction with hemorrhagic change.

Diagnosis

- Posterior cerebral artery infarct

Chapter 6

Spinal Cord

 Key Concepts

1) The adult spinal cord terminates (conus terminalis) at the lower border of the first lumbar vertebra.
2) The newborn's spinal cord extends to the third lumbar vertebra. In adults, the cauda equina extends from vertebral level L-2 to coccygeal vertebra (Co).

I GRAY AND WHITE RAMI COMMUNICANS (Figure 6-1)

A. Gray rami communicans contain unmyelinated postganglionic sympathetic fibers. They are found at all levels of the spinal cord.

B. White rami communicans contain myelinated preganglionic sympathetic fibers. They are found from T-1 to L-3 (the extent of the lateral horn and the intermediolateral cell column).

II TERMINATION OF THE CONUS MEDULLARIS (see Figure 4-1) occurs in the newborn at the level of the body of the third lumbar vertebra (L-3). In the adult, it occurs at the level of the lower border of the first lumbar vertebra (L-1). This is clinically relevant in determining the appropriate position for performing lumbar puncture in children and adults.

III LOCATION OF THE MAJOR MOTOR AND SENSORY NUCLEI OF THE SPINAL CORD (Figure 6-2)

A. The **ciliospinal center of Budge**, from C-8 to T-2, mediates the sympathetic innervation of the eye.

B. The **intermediolateral nucleus (cell column)** of the lateral horn, from C-8 to L-3, mediates the entire sympathetic innervation of the body.

C. The **nucleus dorsalis of Clark**, from C-8 to L-3, gives rise to the dorsal spinocerebellar tract.

D. The **sacral parasympathetic nucleus**, from S-2 to S-4

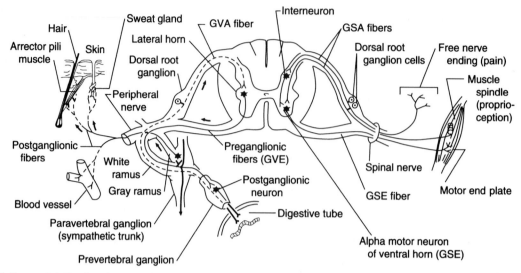

● **Figure 6-1** The four functional components of the thoracic spinal nerve: general visceral afferent (*GVA*), general somatic afferent (*GSA*), general somatic efferent (*GSE*), and general visceral efferent (*GVE*). Proprioceptive, cutaneous, and visceral reflex arcs are shown. The muscle stretch (myotatic) reflex includes the muscle spindle, GSA dorsal root ganglion cell, GSE ventral horn motor neuron, and skeletal muscle.

    E.   The **nucleus of the accessory nerve**, from C-1 to C-6

    F.   The **phrenic nucleus**, from C-3 to C-6

IV   **THE CAUDA EQUINA**   Motor and sensory roots that are found in the subarachnoid space below the conus medullaris form the cauda equina. They exit the vertebral canal through the lumbar intervertebral and sacral foramina.

V   **THE MYOTATIC REFLEX** (see Figure 6-1) is a monosynaptic and ipsilateral **muscle stretch reflex (MSR)**. Like all reflexes, the myotatic reflex has an afferent and an efferent limb. **Interruption of either limb** results in **areflexia.**

    A.   The **afferent limb** includes a muscle spindle (receptor) and a dorsal root ganglion neuron and its Ia fiber.

    B.   The **efferent limb** includes a ventral horn motor neuron that innervates striated muscle (effector).

    C.   The **five most commonly tested MSRs** are listed in Table 6-1.

TABLE 6-1	THE FIVE MOST COMMONLY TESTED MUSCLE STRETCH REFLEXES	
Muscle Stretch Reflex	**Cord Segment**	**Muscle**
Ankle jerk	S-1	Gastrocnemius
Knee jerk	L-2–L-4	Quadriceps
Biceps jerk	C-5 and C-6	Biceps
Forearm jerk	C-5 and C-6	Brachioradialis
Triceps jerk	C-7 and C-8	Triceps

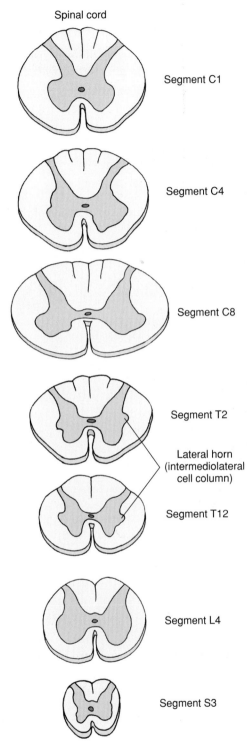

Spinal cord

Segment C1

Segment C4

Segment C8

Segment T2

Lateral horn
(intermediolateral
cell column)

Segment T12

Segment L4

Segment S3

● **Figure 6-2** Spinal cord segments. Cervical segments are the largest segments. The thoracic and sacral segments are relatively small. Note the presence of an intermediolateral cell column in the thoracic and sacral segments. (Reprinted from A Siegel, HN Sapru, *Essential neuroscience*. Baltimore: Lippincott Williams & Wilkins, 2006:142, with permission.)

Case Study

A 46-year-old man was admitted with complaints of lower back pain that radiated down to his foot over the last 2 months. The pain was not relieved with medical therapy. What is your diagnosis?

Relevant Physical Exam Findings

- Absent right ankle jerk
- Weakness of dorsiflexion and plantar flexion
- Decreased pinprick over the dorsum of the foot

Relevant Lab Findings

- An anteroposterior myelogram demonstrated compression of the first sacral nerve root on the left at the level of the L5-S1 vertebrae.

Diagnosis

- Lumbar intervertebral disc herniation

Chapter 7

Autonomic Nervous System

 ## Key Concepts

Understand the etiology of Horner's syndrome. Make sure you know the actions of the autonomic nervous system on the organ systems (Table 7.1).

I   INTRODUCTION   The autonomic nervous system (ANS) is a general visceral efferent motor system that **controls and regulates smooth muscle, cardiac muscle, and glands.**

A. The ANS consists of two types of **projection neurons:**
   1. **Preganglionic neurons.**
   2. **Postganglionic neurons.** Sympathetic ganglia have interneurons.

B. **AUTONOMIC OUTPUT** is controlled by the **hypothalamus.**

C. The ANS has **three divisions:**
   1. **Sympathetic.** Figure 7-1 shows the sympathetic innervation of the ANS.
   2. **Parasympathetic.** Figure 7-2 shows the parasympathetic innervation of the ANS. Table 7-1 compares the effects of sympathetic and parasympathetic activity on organ systems.
   3. **Enteric.** The enteric division includes the intramural ganglia of the gastrointestinal tract, submucosal plexus, and myenteric plexus.

II   CRANIAL NERVES (CN) WITH PARASYMPATHETIC COMPONENTS include the following:

A. **CN III** (ciliary ganglion).

B. **CN VII** (pterygopalatine and submandibular ganglia).

C. **CN IX** (otic ganglion).

D. **CN X** [terminal (intramural) ganglia].

III   COMMUNICATING RAMI of the ANS include the following:

A. **WHITE RAMI COMMUNICANTES,** which are found between T-1 and L-2 and are myelinated.

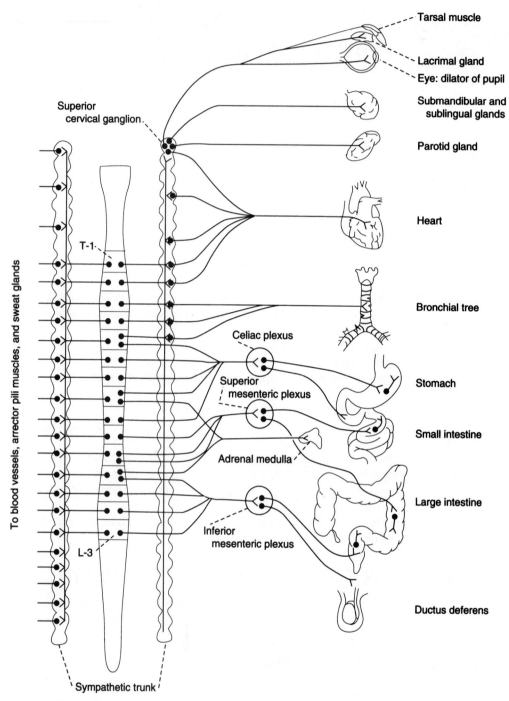

● **Figure 7-1** The sympathetic (thoracolumbar) innervation of the autonomic nervous system. The entire sympathetic innervation of the head is through the superior cervical ganglion. Gray communicating rami are found at all spinal cord levels. White communicating rami are found only in spinal segments T-1 through L-2.

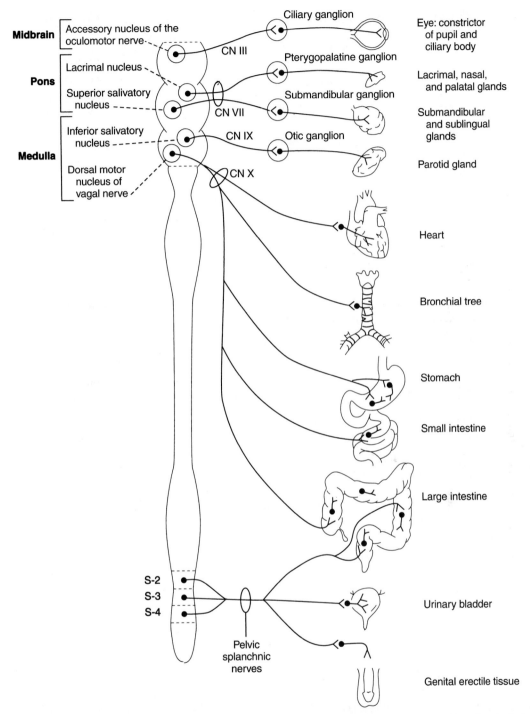

● **Figure 7-2** The parasympathetic (craniosacral) innervation of the autonomic nervous system. Sacral outflow includes segments S-2 through S-4. Cranial outflow is mediated through cranial nerves (*CN*) III, VII, IX, and X.

TABLE 7-1	SYMPATHETIC AND PARASYMPATHETIC ACTIVITY ON ORGAN SYSTEMS	
Structure	Sympathetic Function	Parasympathetic Function
Eye		
Radial muscle of iris	Dilation of pupil (mydriasis)	
Circular muscle of iris		Constriction of pupil (miosis)
Ciliary muscle of ciliary body		Contraction for near vision
Lacrimal gland		Stimulation of secretion
Salivary glands	Viscous secretion	Watery secretion
Sweat glands		
Thermoregulatory	Increase	
Apocrine (stress)	Increase	
Heart		
Sinoatrial node	Acceleration	Deceleration (vagal arrest)
Atrioventricular node	Increase in conduction velocity	Decrease in conduction velocity
Contractility	Increase	Decrease (atria)
Vascular smooth muscle		
Skin, splanchnic vessels	Contraction	
Skeletal muscle vessels	Relaxation	
Bronchiolar smooth muscle	Relaxation	Contraction
Gastrointestinal tract		
Smooth muscle		
Walls	Relaxation	Contraction
Sphincters	Contraction	Relaxation
Secretions and motility	Decrease	Increase
Genitourinary tract		
Smooth muscle		
Bladder wall	Little or no effect	Contraction
Sphincter	Contraction	Relaxation
Penis, seminal vesicles	Ejaculation[a]	Erection[a]
Adrenal medulla	Secretion of epinephrine and norepinephrine	
Metabolic functions		
Liver	Gluconeogenesis and glycogenolysis	
Fat cells	Lipolysis	
Kidney	Renin release	

[a]Note erection versus ejaculation: Remember **p**oint and **s**hoot, where p = parasympathetic and s = sympathetic.
Reprinted from J Fix, *BRS neuroanatomy*. Media, PA: Williams & Wilkins, 1991, with permission.

B. GRAY RAMI COMMUNICANTES, which are found at all spinal levels and are unmyelinated.

IV   NEUROTRANSMITTERS of the ANS include

A. ACETYLCHOLINE, which is the neurotransmitter of the preganglionic neurons.

B. NOREPINEPHRINE, which is the neurotransmitter of the postganglionic neurons, with the exception of sweat glands and some blood vessels that receive cholinergic sympathetic innervation.

C. **DOPAMINE,** which is the neurotransmitter of the small, intensely fluorescent (SIF) cells, which are interneurons of the sympathetic ganglia.

D. **VASOACTIVE INTESTINAL POLYPEPTIDE** (VIP), a vasodilator that is colocalized with acetylcholine in some postganglionic parasympathetic fibers.

E. **NITRIC OXIDE** (NO), a newly discovered neurotransmitter that is responsible for the relaxation of smooth muscle. It is also responsible for penile erection (see Chapter 23).

Ⓥ CLINICAL CORRELATION

A. **MEGACOLON (HIRSCHSPRUNG'S DISEASE,** OR **CONGENITAL AGANGLIONIC MEGACOLON)** is characterized by extreme dilation and hypertrophy of the colon, with fecal retention, and by the absence of ganglion cells in the myenteric plexus. It occurs when neural crest cells do not migrate into the colon.

B. **FAMILIAL DYSAUTONOMIA (RILEY-DAY SYNDROME)** predominantly affects Jewish children. It is an autosomal recessive trait that is characterized by abnormal sweating, unstable blood pressure (e.g., orthostatic hypotension), difficulty in feeding (as a result of inadequate muscle tone in the gastrointestinal tract), and progressive sensory loss. It results in the loss of neurons in the autonomic and sensory ganglia.

C. **RAYNAUD'S DISEASE** is a painful disorder of the terminal arteries of the extremities. It is characterized by idiopathic paroxysmal bilateral cyanosis of the digits (as a result of arterial and arteriolar constriction because of cold or emotion). It may be treated by preganglionic sympathectomy.

D. **PEPTIC ULCER DISEASE** results from excessive production of hydrochloric acid because of increased parasympathetic (tone) stimulation.

E. **HORNER'S SYNDROME** (see Chapter 15) is oculosympathetic paralysis.

F. **SHY-DRAGER SYNDROME** involves preganglionic sympathetic neurons from the intermediolateral cell column. It is characterized by orthostatic hypotension, anhidrosis, impotence, and bladder atonicity.

G. **BOTULISM.** The toxin of *Clostridium botulinum* blocks the release of acetylcholine and results in paralysis of all striated muscles. Autonomic effects include dry eyes, dry mouth, and gastrointestinal ileus (bowel obstruction).

H. **LAMBERT-EATON MYASTHENIC SYNDROME** is a presynaptic disorder of neuromuscular transmission in which acetylcholine release is impaired, resulting in autonomic dysfunction (such as dry mouth) as well as proximal muscle weakness and abnormal tendon reflexes.

Chapter 8

Tracts of the Spinal Cord

 Key Concepts

The most important tracts of the spinal cord are corticospinal (pyramidal), posterior (dorsal) columns, pain and temperature. Know them cold!

I **INTRODUCTION** Figure 8-1 shows the ascending and descending tracts of the spinal cord. This chapter covers four of the major tracts.

II **POSTERIOR (DORSAL) COLUMN—MEDIAL LEMNISCUS PATHWAY** (Figure 8-1 and 8-2; see also Figure 9-1)

A. FUNCTION. The posterior (dorsal) column—medial lemniscus pathway mediates tactile discrimination, vibration sensation, form recognition, and joint and muscle sensation (conscious proprioception).

B. RECEPTORS include Pacinian and Meissner's tactile corpuscles, joint receptors, muscle spindles, and Golgi tendon organs.

C. FIRST-ORDER NEURONS are located in the spinal (dorsal root) ganglia at all levels. They project axons to the spinal cord through the medial root entry zone. First-order neurons give rise to
   1. The gracile fasciculus from the lower extremity.
   2. The cuneate fasciculus from the upper extremity.
   3. The collaterals for spinal reflexes (e.g., myotatic reflex).
   4. The axons that ascend in the dorsal columns and terminate in the gracile and cuneate nuclei of the caudal medulla.

D. SECOND-ORDER NEURONS are located in the gracile and cuneate nuclei of the caudal medulla. They give rise to axons and internal arcuate fibers that decussate and form a compact fiber bundle (i.e., medial lemniscus). The medial lemniscus ascends through the contralateral brain stem and terminates in the ventral posterolateral (VPL) nucleus of the thalamus.

E. THIRD-ORDER NEURONS are located in the VPL nucleus of the thalamus. They project through the posterior limb of the internal capsule to the postcentral gyrus, which is the primary somatosensory cortex (Brodmann's areas 3, 1, and 2).

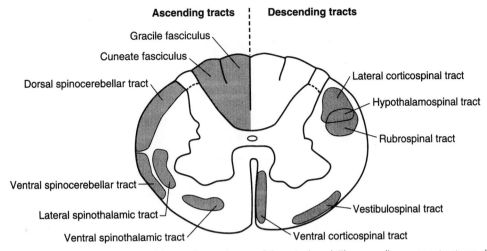

● **Figure 8-1** The major ascending and descending pathways of the spinal cord. The ascending sensory tracts are shown on the left, and the descending motor tracts are shown on the right.

F. TRANSECTION OF THE POSTERIOR (DORSAL) COLUMN–MEDIAL LEMNISCUS TRACT

1. **Above the sensory decussation,** transection results in contralateral loss of the posterior (dorsal) column modalities.

2. **In the spinal cord,** transection results in ipsilateral loss of the posterior (dorsal) column modalities.

III   LATERAL SPINOTHALAMIC TRACT (Figure 8-1 and 8-3; see also Figure 9-1)

A. FUNCTION. The lateral spinothalamic tract mediates pain and temperature sensation.

B. RECEPTORS are free nerve endings. The lateral spinothalamic tract receives input from fast- and slow-conducting pain fibers (i.e., A-δ and C, respectively).

C. FIRST-ORDER NEURONS are found in the spinal (dorsal root) ganglia at all levels. They project axons to the spinal cord through the dorsolateral tract of Lissauer (lateral root entry zone) to second-order neurons.

D. SECOND-ORDER NEURONS are found in the dorsal horn. They give rise to axons that decussate in the **ventral white commissure** and ascend in the contralateral lateral funiculus. Their axons terminate in the VPL nucleus of the thalamus.

E. THIRD-ORDER NEURONS are found in the VPL nucleus of the thalamus. They project through the posterior limb of the internal capsule to the primary somatosensory cortex (Brodmann's areas 3, 1, and 2).

F. TRANSECTION OF THE LATERAL SPINOTHALAMIC TRACT results in contralateral loss of pain and temperature below the lesion.

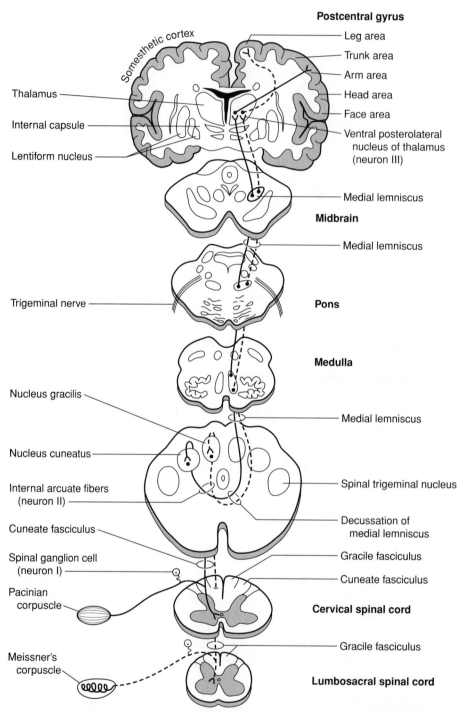

● **Figure 8-2** The dorsal column–medial lemniscus pathway. Impulses conducted by this pathway mediate discriminatory tactile sense (e.g., touch, vibration, pressure) and kinesthetic sense (e.g., position, movement). The posterior (dorsal) column system mediates conscious proprioception. (Adapted from MB Carpenter, J Sutin, *Human neuroanatomy*. Baltimore: Williams & Wilkins, 1983:266, with permission.)

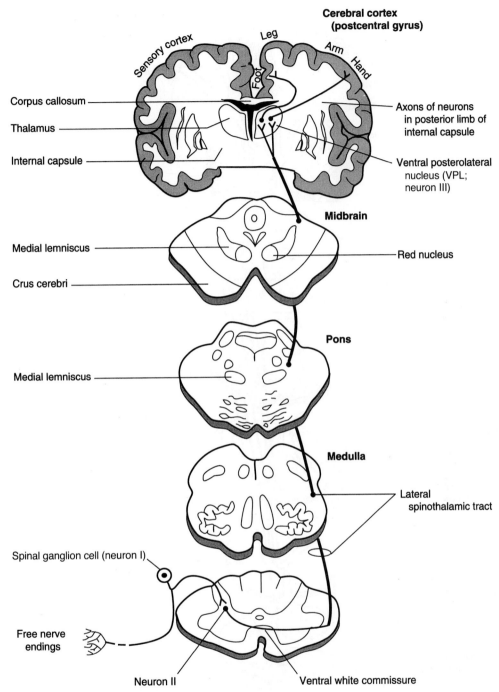

● Figure 8-3 The lateral spinothalamic tract. Impulses conducted by this tract mediate pain and thermal sense. Numerous collaterals are distributed to the brain stem reticular formation. (Adapted from MB Carpenter, J Sutin, *Human neuroanatomy*. Baltimore: Williams & Wilkins, 1983:274, with permission.)

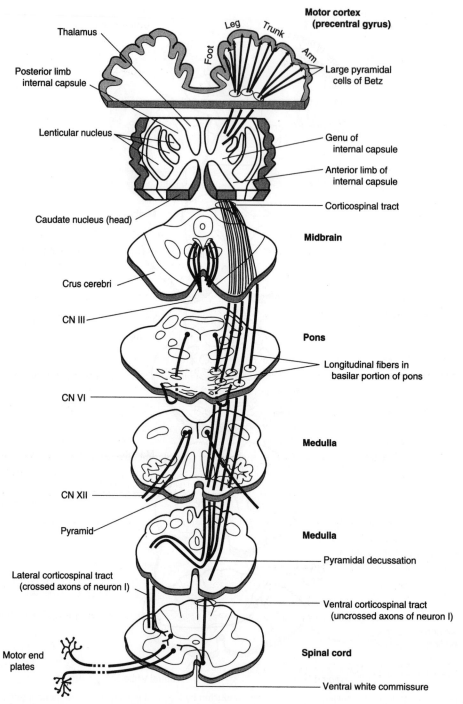

● **Figure 8-4** The lateral and ventral corticospinal (pyramidal) tracts. These major descending motor pathways mediate volitional motor activity. The cells of origin are located in the premotor, the motor, and the sensory cortices. *CN*, cranial nerve. (Adapted from MB Carpenter, J Sutin, *Human neuroanatomy*. Baltimore: Williams & Wilkins, 1983:285, with permission.)

LATERAL CORTICOSPINAL TRACT (Figure 8-1 and 8-4; see also Figure 9-1)

A. FUNCTION. The lateral corticospinal tract mediates voluntary skilled motor activity, primarily of the upper limbs. It is not fully myelinated until the end of the second year (Babinski's sign).

B. FIBER CALIBER. Approximately 90% of the fibers lie between 1 and 4 μ, and 4% lie above 20 μm (from the giant cells of Betz).

C. ORIGIN AND TERMINATION
   1. Origin. The lateral corticospinal tract arises from layer V of the cerebral cortex from three cortical areas in equal aliquots:
      a. The **premotor cortex** (Brodmann's area 6).
      b. The **primary motor cortex,** or precentral gyrus (Brodmann's area 4).
      Arm, face, and foot areas. The arm and face areas of the motor homunculus arise from the lateral convexity; the foot region of the motor homunculus is found in the paracentral lobule (see Figure 23-2).
      c. The **primary sensory cortex,** or postcentral gyrus (Brodmann's areas 3, 1, and 2).
   2. Termination. The lateral corticospinal tract terminates contralaterally, through interneurons, on ventral horn motor neurons.

D. COURSE of the lateral corticospinal tract
   1. Telencephalon. The lateral corticospinal tract runs in the posterior limb of the internal capsule in the telencephalon.
   2. Midbrain. The lateral corticospinal tract runs in the middle three-fifths of the crus cerebri in the midbrain.
   3. Pons. The lateral corticospinal tract runs in the base of the pons.
   4. Medulla. The lateral corticospinal tract runs in the medullary pyramids. Between 85% and 90% of the corticospinal fibers cross in the pyramidal decussation as the lateral corticospinal tract. The remaining 10% to 15% of the fibers continue as the anterior corticospinal tract.
   5. Spinal cord. The lateral corticospinal tract runs in the dorsal quadrant of the lateral funiculus.

E. TRANSECTION OF THE LATERAL CORTICOSPINAL TRACT
   1. Above the motor decussation, transection results in contralateral spastic paresis and Babinski's sign (upward fanning of the toes).
   2. In the spinal cord, transection results in ipsilateral spastic paresis and Babinski's sign.

HYPOTHALAMOSPINAL TRACT (Figure 8-5)

A. ANATOMIC LOCATION. The hypothalamospinal tract projects without interruption from the hypothalamus to the ciliospinal center of the intermediolateral cell column at T-1 to T-2. It is found in the spinal cord at T-1 or above in the dorsolateral quadrant of the lateral funiculus. It is also found in the lateral tegmentum of the medulla, pons, and midbrain.

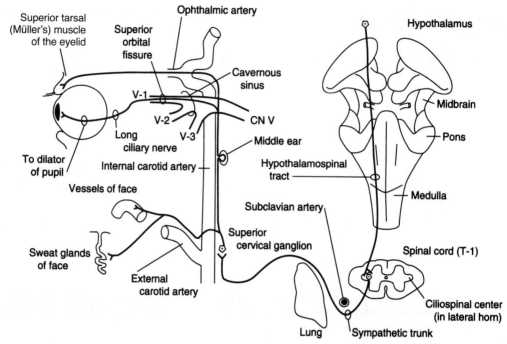

● **Figure 8-5** The oculosympathetic pathway. Hypothalamic fibers project to the ipsilateral ciliospinal center of the inter-mediolateral cell column at T-1. The ciliospinal center projects preganglionic sympathetic fibers to the superior cervical ganglion. The superior cervical ganglion projects perivascular postganglionic sympathetic fibers through the tympanic cavity, cavernous sinus, and superior orbital fissure to the dilator muscle of the iris. Interruption of this pathway at any level results in Horner's syndrome. *CN,* cranial nerve.

B. CLINICAL FEATURES. Interruption of this tract at any level results in Horner's syndrome (i.e., miosis, ptosis, hemianhidrosis, and apparent enophthalmos). The signs are always ipsilateral.

Case Study

A 17-year-old man complained of pain on the left side of his chest and progressive weakness of his left lower limb for 2 months before coming to the clinic. What is the most likely diagnosis?

Relevant Physical Exam Findings

- Neurologic evaluation revealed weakness in the left lower limb; spasticity and hyper-reflexia at the knee and ankle were also observed.
- On the left side, a loss of two-point discrimination, vibratory sense, and proprioception below the hip was observed. A loss of pain and temperature sensation below the T7 dermatome was observed on the right side.

Diagnosis

- Brown-Séquard syndrome, resulting from an upper motor neuron lesion (tumor) at T5-T6 spinal cord levels, represents an incomplete spinal cord lesion characterized by symptoms indicative of hemisection of the spinal cord. It involves ipsilateral hemiplegia with contralateral pain and temperature deficits due to decussating fibers of the spinothalamic tract.

Chapter 9

Lesions of the Spinal Cord

 Key Concepts

Study the eight classic national board lesions of the spinal cord. Four heavy hitters are Brown-Siquard syndrome, B_{12} avitaminosis (subacute combined degeneration), syringomyelia, and amyotrophic lateral sclerosis (ALS, or Lou Gehrig's disease).

I ## DISEASES OF THE MOTOR NEURONS AND CORTICOSPINAL TRACTS
(Figures 9-1 and 9-2)

A. **UPPER MOTOR NEURON (UMN) LESIONS ARE CAUSED BY TRANSECTION OF THE CORTICOSPINAL TRACT OR DESTRUCTION OF THE CORTICAL CELLS OF ORIGIN. THEY RESULT IN SPASTIC PARESIS** with pyramidal signs (Babinski's sign).

B. **LOWER MOTOR NEURON (LMN) LESIONS ARE CAUSED BY DAMAGE TO THE MOTOR NEURONS. THEY RESULT IN FLACCID PARALYSIS,** areflexia, atrophy, fasciculations, and fibrillations. **Poliomyelitis** or Werdnig-Hoffmann disease (Figure 9-2A) results from damage to the motor neurons.

C. An example of a combined UMN and LMN disease is amyotrophic lateral sclerosis (ALS, or Lou Gehrig's disease) (Figure 9-2D). ALS is caused by damage to the corticospinal tracts, with pyramidal signs, and by damage to the LMNs, with LMN symptoms. Patients with ALS have no sensory deficits.

II ## SENSORY PATHWAY LESIONS   An example of a condition caused by these lesions is **dorsal column disease (tabes dorsalis)** (Figure 9-2C). This disease is seen in patients with neurosyphilis. It is characterized by a loss of tactile discrimination and position and vibration sensation. Irritative involvement of the dorsal roots results in pain and paresthesias. Patients have a Romberg sign. (Subject stands with his feet together and, when he closes his eyes, loses his balance. This is a sign of dorsal column ataxia.)

III ## COMBINED MOTOR AND SENSORY LESIONS

A. **SPINAL CORD HEMISECTION (BROWN-SÉQUARD SYNDROME)** (Figure 9-2E) is caused by damage to the following structures:
   1. The **dorsal columns [gracile (leg) and cuneate (arm) fasciculi].** Damage results in ipsilateral loss of tactile discrimination and position and vibration sensation.

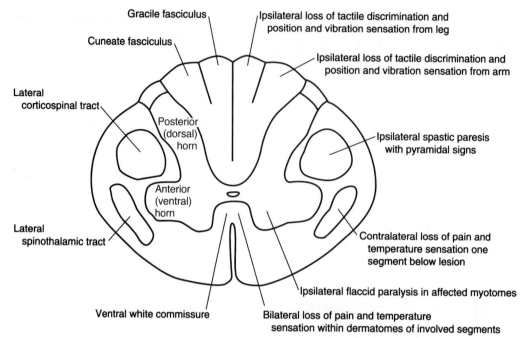

● **Figure 9-1** Transverse section of the cervical spinal cord. The clinically important ascending and descending pathways are shown on the left. Clinical deficits that result from the interruption of these pathways are shown on the right. Destructive lesions of the posterior (dorsal) horns result in anesthesia and areflexia. Destruction of the ventral white commissure interrupts the central transmission of pain and temperature impulses bilaterally through the lateral spinothalamic tracts.

2. The **lateral corticospinal tract.** Damage results in ipsilateral spastic paresis with pyramidal signs below the lesion.
3. The **lateral spinothalamic tract.** Damage results in contralateral loss of pain and temperature sensation one segment below the lesion.
4. The **hypothalamospinal tract at T-1 and above.** Damage results in ipsilateral Horner's syndrome (i.e., miosis, ptosis, hemianhidrosis, and apparent enophthalmos).
5. The **ventral (anterior) horn.** Damage results in ipsilateral flaccid paralysis of innervated muscles.

B. **VENTRAL SPINAL ARTERY OCCLUSION** (Figure 9-2F) causes infarction of the anterior two-thirds of the spinal cord but spares the dorsal columns and horns. It results in damage to the following structures:
1. The **lateral corticospinal tracts.** Damage results in bilateral spastic paresis with pyramidal signs below the lesion.
2. The **lateral spinothalamic tracts.** Damage results in bilateral loss of pain and temperature sensation below the lesion.
3. The **hypothalamospinal tract at T-2 and above.** Damage results in bilateral Horner's syndrome.
4. The **ventral (anterior) horns.** Damage results in bilateral flaccid paralysis of the innervated muscles.
5. The **corticospinal tracts to the sacral parasympathetic centers at S-2 to S-4.** Damage results in bilateral damage and loss of voluntary bladder and bowel control.

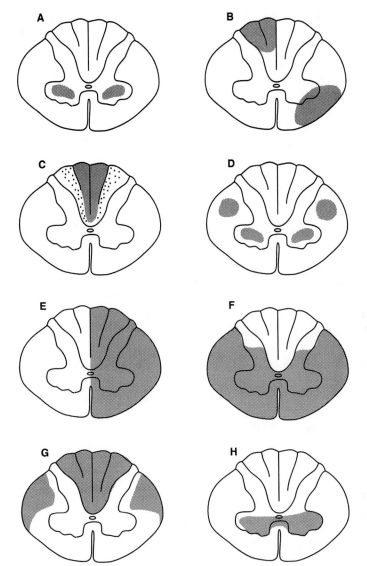

● **Figure 9-2** Classic lesions of the spinal cord. **(A)** Poliomyelitis and progressive infantile muscular atrophy (Werdnig-Hoffmann disease). **(B)** Multiple sclerosis. **(C)** Posterior (dorsal) column disease (tabes dorsalis). **(D)** Amyotrophic lateral sclerosis. **(E)** Hemisection of the spinal cord (Brown-Séquard syndrome). **(F)** Complete anterior (ventral) spinal artery occlusion of the spinal cord. **(G)** Subacute combined degeneration (vitamin B$_{12}$ neuropathy). **(H)** Syringomyelia.

C. SUBACUTE COMBINED DEGENERATION (VITAMIN B$_{12}$ NEUROPATHY) (Figure 9-2G) is caused by pernicious (megaloblastic) anemia. It results from damage to the following structures:

1. The **dorsal columns (gracile and cuneate fasciculi)**. Damage results in bilateral loss of tactile discrimination and position and vibration sensation.

2. The **lateral corticospinal tracts**. Damage results in bilateral spastic paresis with pyramidal signs.

3. The **spinocerebellar tracts**. Damage results in bilateral arm and leg dystaxia.

D. SYRINGOMYELIA (Figure 9-2H) is a central cavitation of the cervical cord of unknown etiology. It results in damage to the following structures:

1. The **ventral white commissure**. Damage to decussating lateral spinothalamic axons causes bilateral loss of pain and temperature sensation.
2. The **ventral horns**. LMN lesions result in flaccid paralysis of the intrinsic muscles of the hands.

E. FRIEDREICH'S ATAXIA HAS THE SAME SPINAL CORD PATHOLOGY AND SYMPTOMS AS SUBACUTE COMBINED DEGENERATION.

F. In **multiple sclerosis** (see Figure 9-2B), the plaques primarily involve the white matter of the cervical segments of the spinal cord. The lesions are random and asymmetric.

IV **PERIPHERAL NERVOUS SYSTEM (PNS) LESIONS** An example of a PNS lesion is **Guillain-Barré syndrome** (acute idiopathic polyneuritis, or postinfectious polyneuritis). It primarily affects the motor fibers of the ventral roots and peripheral nerves, and it produces LMN symptoms (i.e., muscle weakness, ascending flaccid paralysis, and areflexia.) Guillain-Barré syndrome has the following features:

A. It is characterized by demyelination and edema.

B. Upper cervical root (C4) involvement and respiratory paralysis are common.

C. Caudal cranial nerve involvement with facial diplegia is present in 50% of cases.

D. Elevated protein levels may cause papilledema.

E. To a lesser degree, sensory fibers are affected, resulting in paresthesias.

F. The protein level in the cerebrospinal fluid is elevated but without pleocytosis (**albuminocytologic dissociation**).

V **INTERVERTEBRAL DISK HERNIATION** is seen at the L-4 to L-5 or L-5 to S-1 interspace in 90% of cases. It appears at the C-5 to C-6 or C-6 to C-7 interspace in 10% of cases.

A. Intervertebral disk herniation consists of prolapse, or herniation, of the **nucleus pulposus through the defective anulus fibrosus and into the vertebral canal.**

B. The nucleus pulposus **impinges on the spinal roots,** resulting in spinal root symptoms (i.e., paresthesias, pain, sensory loss, hyporeflexia, and muscle weakness).

VI **CAUDA EQUINA SYNDROME (SPINAL ROOTS L3 TO CO)** results usually from a nerve root tumor, an ependymoma, or a dermoid tumor, or from a lipoma of the terminal cord. It is characterized by

A. Severe radicular unilateral pain.

B. Sensory distribution in a unilateral **saddle-shaped** area.

C. Unilateral muscle atrophy and absent quadriceps (L3) and ankle jerks (S1).

D. Unremarkable incontinence and sexual functions.

E. Gradual and unilateral onset.

VII   CONUS MEDULLARIS SYNDROME (CORD SEGMENTS S3 TO CO) usually results from an intramedullary tumor (e.g., ependymoma). It is characterized by

A. Pain, usually bilateral and not severe.

B. Sensory distribution in a bilateral **saddle-shaped** area.

C. Unremarkable muscle changes; normal quadriceps and ankle reflexes.

D. Severely impaired incontinence and sexual functions.

E. Sudden and bilateral onset.

Chapter 10

Brain Stem

Key Concepts

1) Study the transverse sections of the brain stem and localize the cranial nerve nuclei.
2) Study the ventral surface of the brain stem and identify the exiting and entering cranial nerves.
3) On the dorsal surface of the brain stem, identify the only exiting cranial nerve, the trochlear nerve.

Ⅰ **INTRODUCTION** The brain stem includes the **medulla, pons,** and **midbrain**. It extends from the pyramidal decussation to the posterior commissure. The brain stem receives its blood supply from the vertebrobasilar system. It contains cranial nerves (CN) III to XII (except the spinal part of CN XI). Figures 10-1 and 10-2 show its surface anatomy.

Ⅱ **CROSS SECTION THROUGH THE MEDULLA** (Figure 10-3)

A. MEDIAL STRUCTURES
1. The **hypoglossal nucleus of CN XII**
2. The **medial lemniscus,** which contains crossed fibers from the gracile and cuneate nuclei
3. The **pyramid** (corticospinal fibers)

B. LATERAL STRUCTURES
1. The **nucleus ambiguus (CN IX, X, and XI)**
2. The **vestibular nuclei (CN VIII)**
3. The **inferior cerebellar peduncle,** which contains the dorsal spinocerebellar, cuneocerebellar, and olivocerebellar tracts
4. The **lateral spinothalamic tract** (spinal lemniscus)
5. The **spinal nucleus** and **tract of trigeminal nerve**

Ⅲ **CROSS SECTION THROUGH THE PONS** (Figure 10-4). The pons has a dorsal tegmentum and a ventral base.

A. MEDIAL STRUCTURES
1. Medial longitudinal fasciculus (MLF)
2. Abducent nucleus of CN VI (underlies facial colliculus)
3. Genu (internal) of CN VII (underlies facial nerve) (facial colliculus)

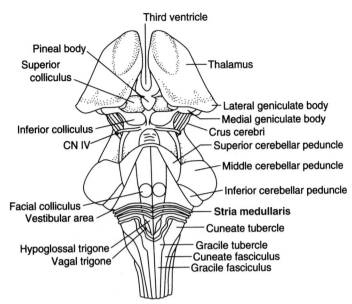

● **Figure 10-1** The dorsal surface of the brain stem. The three cerebellar peduncles have been removed to expose the rhomboid fossa. The trochlear nerve is the only nerve to exit the brain stem from the dorsal surface. The facial colliculus surmounts the genu of the facial nerve and the abducent nucleus. *CN,* cranial nerve.

4. Abducent fibers of CN VI
5. Medial lemniscus
6. Corticospinal tract (in the base of the pons)

B. LATERAL STRUCTURES
1. Facial nucleus (CN VII)
2. Facial (intraaxial) nerve fibers
3. Spinal nucleus and tract of trigeminal nerve (CN V)

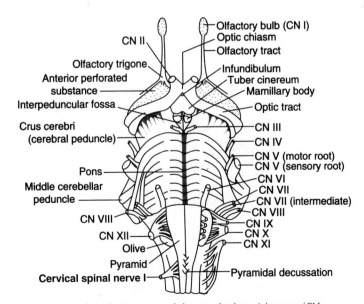

● **Figure 10-2** The ventral surface of the brain stem and the attached cranial nerves (*CN*).

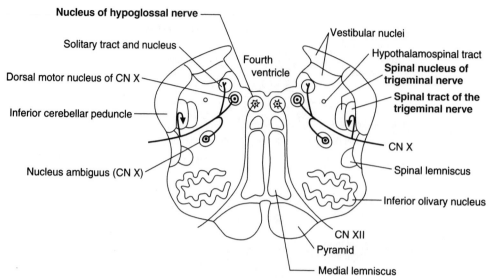

● **Figure 10-3** Transverse section of the medulla at the midolivary level. The vagal nerve [cranial nerve (*CN*) X], hypoglossal nerve (CN XII), and vestibulocochlear nerve (CN VIII) are prominent in this section. The nucleus ambiguus gives rise to special visceral efferent fibers to CN IX, X, and XI.

4. Lateral spinothalamic tract (spinal lemniscus)
5. Vestibular nuclei of CN VIII
6. Cochlear nuclei of CN VIII

 IV **CROSS SECTION THROUGH THE ROSTRAL MIDBRAIN** (Figure 10-5). The midbrain has a dorsal tectum, an intermediate tegmentum, and a base. The aqueduct lies between the tectum and the tegmentum.

A. DORSAL STRUCTURES include the **superior colliculi.**

B. TEGMENTUM
   1. Oculomotor nucleus (CN III)
   2. Medial longitudinal fasciculus (MLF)

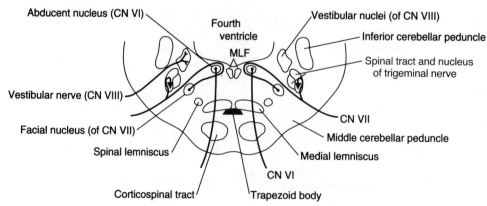

● **Figure 10-4** Transverse section of the pons at the level of the abducent nucleus of cranial nerve (*CN*) VI and the facial nucleus of CN VII. *MLF*, medial longitudinal fasciculus.

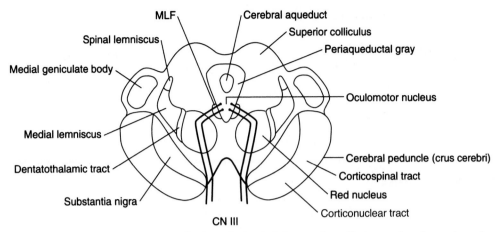

● **Figure 10-5** Transverse section of the midbrain at the level of the superior colliculus, oculomotor nucleus of cranial nerve (*CN*) III, and red nucleus. *MLF*, medial longitudinal fasciculus.

3. Red nucleus
4. Substantia nigra
5. Dentatothalamic tract (crossed)
6. Medial lemniscus
7. Lateral spinothalamic tract (in the spinal lemniscus)

C. **CRUS CEREBRI** (basis pedunculi cerebri, or cerebral peduncle). The **corticospinal tract** lies in the middle three-fifths of the crus cerebri.

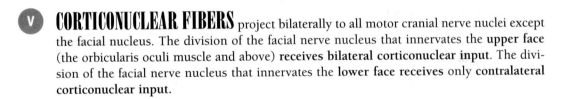

CORTICONUCLEAR FIBERS project bilaterally to all motor cranial nerve nuclei except the facial nucleus. The division of the facial nerve nucleus that innervates the **upper face** (the orbicularis oculi muscle and above) **receives bilateral corticonuclear input**. The division of the facial nerve nucleus that innervates the **lower face receives** only **contralateral corticonuclear input**.

Chapter 11

Cranial Nerves

✔ Key Concepts

1) This chapter is pivotal. It spawns more neuroanatomy examination questions than any other chapter. Carefully study all of the figures and legends.
2) The seventh cranial nerve deserves special consideration (see Figures 11-5 and 11-6). Understand the difference between an upper motor neuron and a lower motor neuron (Bell's palsy).

 THE OLFACTORY NERVE, the first cranial nerve **(CN I)** (Figure 11-1), mediates olfaction **(smell).** It is the only sensory system that has no precortical relay in the thalamus. The olfactory nerve is a special visceral afferent (SVA) nerve; see Appendix I. It consists of unmyelinated axons of bipolar neurons that are located in the nasal mucosa, the olfactory epithelium. It enters the cranial cavity through the **cribriform plate of the ethmoid bone** (see Appendix I).

A. OLFACTORY PATHWAY
1. **Olfactory receptor cells** are first-order neurons that project to the mitral cells of the olfactory bulb.
2. **Mitral cells** are the principal cells of the olfactory bulb. They are excitatory and glutaminergic. They project through the **olfactory tract** and **lateral olfactory stria** to the primary olfactory cortex and amygdala.
3. **The primary olfactory cortex (Brodmann's area 34)** consists of the piriform cortex that overlies the uncus.

B. LESIONS OF THE OLFACTORY PATHWAY result from trauma (e.g., skull fracture) and often from olfactory groove meningiomas. These lesions cause **ipsilateral anosmia** (localizing value). Lesions that involve the parahippocampal uncus may cause olfactory hallucinations [uncinate fits (seizures) with déjà vu].

C. FOSTER KENNEDY SYNDROME consists of ipsilateral anosmia, ipsilateral optic atrophy, and contralateral papilledema. It is usually caused by an anterior fossa meningioma.

THE OPTIC NERVE (CN II) is a special somatic afferent (SSA) nerve that subserves vision and pupillary light reflexes (afferent limb; see Chapter 15). It enters the cranial cavity through the optic canal of the sphenoid bone. It is **not a true peripheral nerve** but is a tract of the diencephalon. A transected optic nerve cannot regenerate.

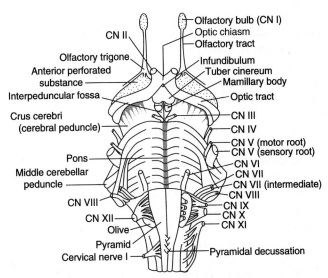

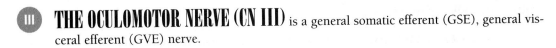

● **Figure 11-1** The base of the brain with attached cranial nerves (*CN*). (Reprinted from RC Truex, CE Kellner. *Detailed atlas of the head and neck*. New York: Oxford University Press, 1958:34, with permission.)

THE OCULOMOTOR NERVE (CN III) is a general somatic efferent (GSE), general visceral efferent (GVE) nerve.

A. GENERAL CHARACTERISTICS. The oculomotor nerve **moves** the **eye, constricts** the **pupil, accommodates,** and **converges.** It exits the brain stem from the interpeduncular fossa of the midbrain, passes through the cavernous sinus, and enters the orbit through the superior orbital fissure.

    1. The **GSE component** arises from the oculomotor nucleus of the rostral midbrain. It innervates four extraocular muscles and the levator palpebrae muscle. (**Remember** the mnemonic SIN: superior muscles are intorters of the globe.)

        a. The **medial rectus muscle** adducts the eye. With its opposite partner, it converges the eyes.

        b. The **superior rectus muscle** elevates, intorts, and adducts the eye.

        c. The **inferior rectus muscle** depresses, extorts, and adducts the eye.

        d. The **inferior oblique muscle** elevates, extorts, and abducts the eye.

        e. The **levator palpebrae muscle** elevates the upper eyelid.

    2. The **GVE component** consists of preganglionic parasympathetic fibers.

        a. The **accessory nucleus of the oculomotor nerve (Edinger-Westphal nucleus)** projects preganglionic parasympathetic fibers to the ciliary ganglion of the orbit through CN III.

        b. The **ciliary ganglion** projects postganglionic parasympathetic fibers to the sphincter pupillae (miosis) and the ciliary muscle (accommodation).

B. CLINICAL CORRELATION

    1. Oculomotor paralysis (palsy) is seen with transtentorial herniation (e.g., tumor, subdural or epidural hematoma).

        a. Denervation of the **levator palpebrae muscle** causes **ptosis** (i.e., drooping of the upper eyelid).

        b. Denervation of the **extraocular muscles** innervated by CN III causes the affected eye to look "down and out" as a result of the unopposed action of the lateral rectus and superior oblique muscles. The superior oblique and lateral rectus muscles are innervated by CN IV and CN VI, respectively. Oculomotor palsy results in **diplopia** (double vision) when the patient looks in the direction of the paretic muscle.

    c. **Interruption of parasympathetic innervation** (internal ophthalmoplegia) results in a **dilated, fixed pupil** and **paralysis of accommodation** (cycloplegia).

  2. **Other conditions associated with CN III impairment**

    a. **Transtentorial (uncal) herniation.** Increased supratentorial pressure (e.g., from a tumor) forces the hippocampal uncus through the tentorial notch and compresses or stretches the oculomotor nerve.

      (1) **Sphincter pupillae fibers** are affected first, resulting in a **dilated, fixed pupil.**

      (2) **Somatic efferent fibers** are affected later, resulting in **external strabismus** (exotropia).

    b. **Aneurysms** of the carotid and posterior communicating arteries often compress CN III within the cavernous sinus or interpeduncular cistern. They usually affect the peripheral pupilloconstrictor fibers first (e.g., uncal herniation).

    c. **Diabetes mellitus (diabetic oculomotor palsy)** often affects the oculomotor nerve. It damages the central fibers and spares the sphincter pupillae fibers.

IV   THE TROCHLEAR NERVE (CN IV) is a GSE nerve.

  A. **GENERAL CHARACTERISTICS.** The trochlear nerve is a pure motor nerve that innervates the superior oblique muscle. This muscle depresses, intorts, and abducts the eye. (Figure 11-2.)

    1. It **arises from** the contralateral trochlear nucleus of the caudal midbrain.

    2. It **decussates** beneath the superior medullary velum of the midbrain and exits the brain stem on its dorsal surface, caudal to the inferior colliculus.

    3. It **encircles the midbrain** within the subarachnoid space, passes through the cavernous sinus, and enters the orbit through the superior orbital fissure.

  B. **CLINICAL CORRELATION.** Because of its course around the midbrain, the trochlear nerve is particularly vulnerable to head trauma. The trochlear decussation underlies the superior medullary velum. Trauma at this site often results in bilateral fourth-nerve palsies. Pressure against the free border of the tentorium (herniation) may injure the nerve (Figure 11-2). **CN IV paralysis** results in the following conditions:

    1. **Extorsion of the eye** and weakness of downward gaze.

    2. **Vertical diplopia,** which increases when looking down.

    3. **Head tilting** to compensate for extorsion (may be misdiagnosed as idiopathic torticollis).

V   THE TRIGEMINAL NERVE (CN V) is a special visceral efferent (SVE), general somatic afferent (GSA) nerve (Figure 11-3).

  A. **GENERAL CHARACTERISTICS.** The trigeminal nerve is the nerve of pharyngeal (branchial) arch 1 (mandibular). It has three divisions: ophthalmic (CN V-1), maxillary (CN V-2), and mandibular (CN V-3).

    1. The **SVE component** arises from the motor nucleus of trigeminal nerve that is found in the lateral midpontine tegmentum. It **innervates** the **muscles of mastication** (i.e.,

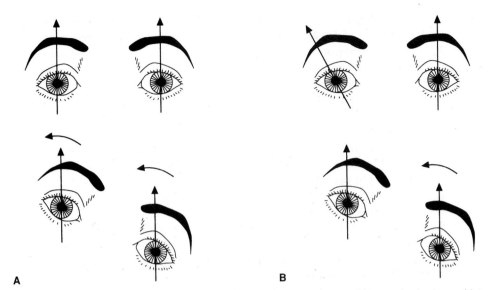

A   **B**

● **Figure 11-2** Paralysis of the right superior oblique muscle. **(A)** A pair of eyes with normal extorsion and intorsion movements. Tilting the chin to the right side results in compensatory intorsion of the left eye and extorsion of the right eye. **(B)** Paralysis of the right superior oblique muscle results in extorsion of the right eye, causing diplopia. Tilting the chin to the right side results in compensatory intorsion of the left eye, thus permitting binocular alignment. (Reprinted from JD Fix. *BRS neuroanatomy*, 3rd ed. Baltimore: Williams & Wilkins, 1996:220, with permission.)

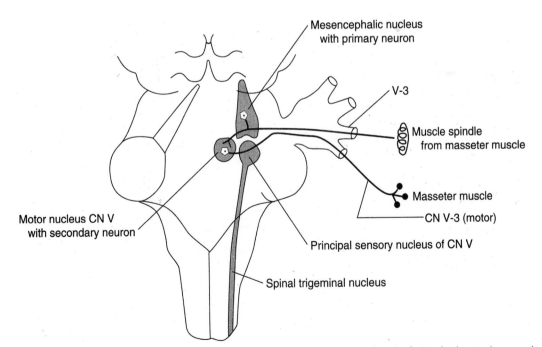

● **Figure 11-3** Jaw jerk (masseter reflex) pathway showing two neurons. Note that the first-order (sensory) neuron is found in the mesencephalic nucleus of the pons and midbrain, not in the trigeminal ganglion. *CN*, cranial nerve. (Reprinted from JD Fix. *BRS neuroanatomy*, 3rd ed. Baltimore: Williams & Wilkins, 1996:220, with permission.)

temporalis, masseter, lateral, and medial pterygoids), the tensors tympani and veli palatini, the mylohyoid muscle, and the anterior belly of the digastric muscle.

2. The **GSA component** provides **sensory innervation to the face,** mucous membranes of the nasal and oral cavities and frontal sinus, hard palate, and deep structures of the head (proprioception from muscles and the temporomandibular joint). It innervates the dura of the anterior and middle cranial fossae (supratentorial dura).

B. **CLINICAL CORRELATION.** Lesions result in the following neurologic deficits:
   1. **Loss of general sensation (hemianesthesia)** from the face and mucous membranes of the oral and nasal cavities.
   2. **Loss of the corneal reflex** (afferent limb, CN V-1; Figure 11-4).
   3. **Flaccid paralysis** of the muscles of mastication.
   4. **Deviation of the jaw to the weak side** as a result of the unopposed action of the opposite lateral pterygoid muscle.
   5. **Paralysis of the tensor tympani muscle,** which leads to hypoacusis (partial deafness to low-pitched sounds).
   6. **Trigeminal neuralgia** (tic douloureux), which is characterized by recurrent paroxysms of sharp, stabbing pain in one or more branches of the nerve.

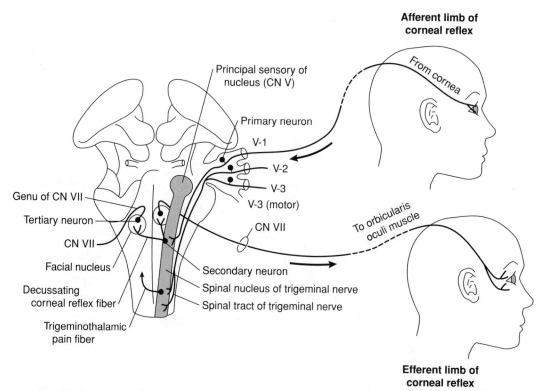

● **Figure 11-4** The corneal reflex pathway showing the three neurons and decussation. This reflex is consensual, like the pupillary light reflex. Second-order pain neurons are found in the caudal division of the spinal nucleus of trigeminal nerve. Second-order corneal reflex neurons are found at more rostral levels. *CN,* cranial nerve.

VI THE ABDUCENT NERVE (CN VI)

A. GENERAL CHARACTERISTICS. The abducent nerve is a pure **GSE nerve** that innervates the lateral rectus muscle, which abducts the eye.

1. It arises from the abducent nucleus that is found in the dorsomedial tegmentum of the caudal pons.
2. Exiting intraaxial fibers pass through the corticospinal tract. A **lesion** results in **alternating abducent hemiparesis.**
3. It passes through the pontine cistern and cavernous sinus and enters the orbit through the superior orbital fissure.

B. CLINICAL CORRELATION. CN VI PARALYSIS is the most common isolated palsy that results from the long peripheral course of the nerve. It is seen in patients with meningitis, subarachnoid hemorrhage, late-stage syphilis, and trauma. **Abducent nerve paralysis** results in the **following defects:**

1. **Convergent (medial) strabismus (esotropia)** with inability to abduct the eye.
2. **Horizontal diplopia** with maximum separation of the double images when looking toward the paretic lateral rectus muscle.

VII THE FACIAL NERVE (CN VII)

A. GENERAL CHARACTERISTICS. The facial nerve is a GSA, general visceral afferent (GVA), SVA, GVE, and SVE nerve (Figures 11-5 and 11-6). It **mediates facial movements, taste, salivation, lacrimation,** and **general sensation from the external ear.** It is the nerve of the pharyngeal (branchial) arch 2 (hyoid). It includes the facial nerve proper (motor division), which contains the SVE fibers that **innervate the muscles of facial (mimetic) expression.** CN VII includes the intermediate nerve, which contains

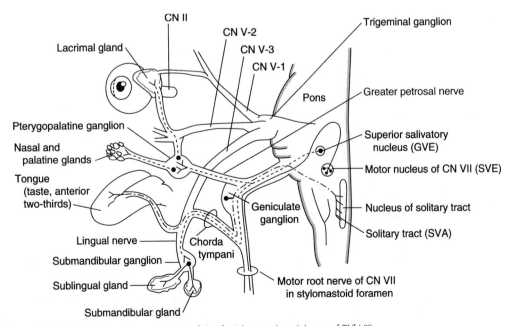

● **Figure 11-5** The functional components of the facial nerve (cranial nerve [*CN*] VII).

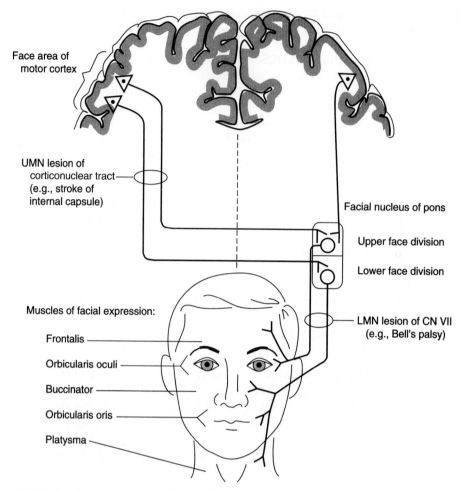

Face area of motor cortex

UMN lesion of corticonuclear tract (e.g., stroke of internal capsule)

Facial nucleus of pons

Upper face division

Lower face division

Muscles of facial expression:

LMN lesion of CN VII (e.g., Bell's palsy)

Frontalis

Orbicularis oculi

Buccinator

Orbicularis oris

Platysma

● **Figure 11-6** Corticonuclear innervation of the facial nerve (cranial nerve [*CN*] VII) nucleus. An upper motor neuron (*UMN*) lesion (e.g., stroke involving the internal capsule) results in contralateral weakness of the lower face, with sparing of the upper face. A lower motor neuron (*LMN*) lesion (e.g., Bell's palsy) results in paralysis of the facial muscles in both the upper and lower face. (Redrawn from WE DeMyer, *Technique of the neurological examination: A programmed text*, 4th ed. New York: McGraw-Hill, 1994:177, with permission.)

GSA, SVA, and GVE fibers. All first-order sensory neurons are found in the geniculate ganglion within the temporal bone.

1. **Anatomy.** The facial nerve exits the brain stem in the cerebellopontine angle. It enters the internal auditory meatus and the facial canal. It then exits the facial canal and skull through the stylomastoid foramen.

2. **The GSA component** has cell bodies located in the geniculate ganglion. It innervates the posterior surface of the external ear through the posterior auricular branch of CN VII. It projects centrally to the spinal tract and nucleus of trigeminal nerve.

3. **The GVA component** has no clinical significance. The cell bodies are located in the geniculate ganglion. Fibers innervate the soft palate and the adjacent pharyngeal wall.

4. **The SVA component (taste)** has cell bodies located in the geniculate ganglion. It projects centrally to the solitary tract and nucleus. It innervates the taste buds from the anterior two-thirds of the tongue through:
   a. The **intermediate nerve.**
   b. The **chorda tympani,** which is located in the tympanic cavity medial to the tympanic membrane and malleus. It contains the SVA and GVE (parasympathetic) fibers.
   c. The **lingual nerve** (a branch of CN V-3).
   d. The **central gustatory pathway** (see Figure 11-5). Taste fibers from CN VII, CN IX, and CN X project through the solitary tract to the solitary nucleus. The solitary nucleus projects through the central tegmental tract to the ventral posteromedial nucleus (VPM) of the thalamus. The VPM projects to the gustatory cortex of the parietal lobe (parietal operculum).
5. The **GVE component** is a parasympathetic component that innervates the lacrimal, submandibular, and sublingual glands. It contains preganglionic parasympathetic neurons that are located in the superior salivatory nucleus of the caudal pons.
   a. **Lacrimal pathway** (see Figure 11-5). The superior salivatory nucleus projects through the intermediate and greater petrosal nerves to the pterygopalatine (sphenopalatine) ganglion. The pterygopalatine ganglion projects to the lacrimal gland of the orbit.
   b. **Submandibular pathway** (see Figure 11-5). The superior salivatory nucleus projects through the intermediate nerve and chorda tympani to the submandibular ganglion. The submandibular ganglion projects to and innervates the submandibular and sublingual glands.
6. The **SVE component** arises from the facial nucleus, loops around the abducent nucleus of the caudal pons, and exits the brain stem in the cerebellopontine angle. It enters the internal auditory meatus, traverses the facial canal, sends a branch to the stapedius muscle of the middle ear, and exits the skull through the stylomastoid foramen. It innervates the muscles of facial expression, the stylohyoid muscle, the posterior belly of the digastric muscle, and the stapedius muscle.

B. **CLINICAL CORRELATION.** Lesions cause the following conditions:
   1. **Flaccid paralysis** of the **muscles of facial expression** (upper and lower face).
   2. **Loss of the corneal reflex** (efferent limb), which may lead to corneal ulceration.
   3. **Loss of taste** (ageusia-gustatory anesthesia) from the anterior two-thirds of the tongue, which may result from damage to the chorda tympani.
   4. **Hyperacusis** (increased acuity to sounds) as a result of stapedius paralysis.
   5. **Bell's palsy** (peripheral facial paralysis), which is caused by trauma or infection and involves the upper and lower face.
   6. **Crocodile tears syndrome** (lacrimation during eating), which is a result of aberrant regeneration of SVE fibers after trauma.
   7. **Supranuclear (central) facial palsy,** which results in contralateral weakness of the lower face, with sparing of the upper face (see Figure 11-6).
   8. **Bilateral facial nerve palsies,** which occur in Guillain-Barré syndrome.
   9. **Möbius' syndrome,** which consists of congenital facial diplegia (CN VII) and convergent strabismus (CN VI).

THE VESTIBULOCOCHLEAR NERVE (CN VIII) is an SSA nerve. It has two functional divisions: the vestibular nerve, which **maintains equilibrium and balance**, and the cochlear nerve, which **mediates hearing**. It exits the brain stem at the cerebellopontine angle and enters the internal auditory meatus. It is confined to the temporal bone.

A. **VESTIBULAR NERVE** (see Figure 14-1)
   1. **General characteristics**
      a. It is associated functionally with the cerebellum (flocculonodular lobe) and ocular motor nuclei.
      b. It regulates compensatory eye movements.
      c. Its first-order sensory bipolar neurons are located in the vestibular ganglion in the fundus of the internal auditory meatus.
      d. It projects its peripheral processes to the hair cells of the cristae of the semicircular ducts and the hair cells of the utricle and saccule.
      e. It projects its central processes to the four vestibular nuclei of the brain stem and the flocculonodular lobe of the cerebellum.
      f. It conducts efferent fibers to the hair cells from the brain stem.
   2. **Clinical correlation.** Lesions result in **disequilibrium, vertigo,** and **nystagmus**.

B. **COCHLEAR NERVE** (see Figure 13-1)
   1. **General characteristics**
      a. Its first-order sensory bipolar neurons are located in the spiral (cochlear) ganglion of the modiolus of the cochlea, within the temporal bone.
      b. It projects its peripheral processes to the hair cells of the organ of Corti.
      c. It projects its central processes to the dorsal and ventral cochlear nuclei of the brain stem.
      d. It conducts efferent fibers to the hair cells from the brain stem.
   2. **Clinical correlation.** Destructive lesions cause **hearing loss** (sensorineural deafness). Irritative lesions can cause **tinnitus** (ear ringing). An **acoustic neuroma** (schwannoma) is a Schwann cell tumor of the cochlear nerve that causes deafness.

THE GLOSSOPHARYNGEAL NERVE (CN IX) is a GSA, GVA, SVA, SVE, and GVE nerve (Figure 11-7).

A. **GENERAL CHARACTERISTICS.** The glossopharyngeal nerve is primarily a sensory nerve. Along with CN X, CN XI, and CN XII, it **mediates taste, salivation,** and **swallowing**. It **mediates input** from the **carotid sinus,** which contains baroreceptors that monitor arterial blood pressure. It also **mediates input** from the **carotid body,** which contains chemoreceptors that monitor the CO_2 and O_2 concentration of the blood.
   1. **Anatomy.** CN IX is the nerve of pharyngeal (branchial) arch 3. It exits the brain stem (medulla) from the postolivary sulcus with CN X and CN XI. It exits the skull through the jugular foramen with CN X and CN XI.
   2. The **GSA component** innervates part of the external ear and the external auditory meatus through the auricular branch of the vagus nerve. It has cell bodies in the superior ganglion. It projects its central processes to the spinal tract and nucleus of trigeminal nerve.

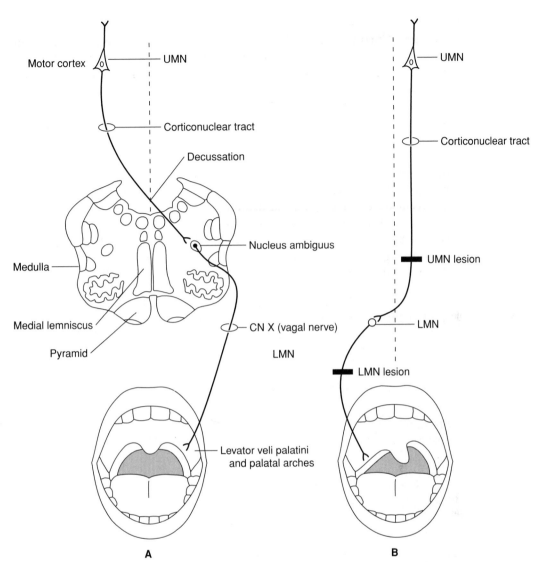

● **Figure 11-7** Innervation of the palatal arches and uvula. Sensory innervation is mediated by the glossopharyngeal nerve [cranial nerve (*CN*) IX]. Motor innervation of the palatal arches and uvula is mediated by the vagus nerve (CN X). **(A)** A normal palate and uvula in a person who is saying "Ah." **(B)** A patient with an upper motor neuron (*UMN*) lesion (left) and a lower motor neuron (*LMN*) lesion (right). When this patient says "Ah," the palatal arches sag. The uvula deviates toward the intact (left) side. (Modified from WE DeMyer, *Technique of the neurological examination: a programmed text*, 4th ed. New York: McGraw-Hill, 1994:191, with permission.)

3. The **GVA component** innervates structures that are derived from the endoderm (e.g., pharynx). It **innervates** the **mucous membranes** of the posterior one-third of the tongue, tonsil, upper pharynx, tympanic cavity, and auditory tube. It also **innervates** the **carotid sinus** (baroreceptors) and **carotid body** (chemoreceptors) through the sinus nerve. It has cell bodies in the inferior (petrosal) ganglion. It is the afferent limb of the gag reflex and the carotid sinus reflex.

4. The **SVA component** innervates the taste buds of the posterior one-third of the tongue. It has cell bodies in the inferior (petrosal) ganglion. It projects its central processes to the solitary tract and nucleus. (For a discussion of the central pathway, see VII.A.4.d.)

5. The SVE **component** innervates only the stylopharyngeus muscle. It arises from the nucleus ambiguus of the lateral medulla.

6. The GVE **component** is a parasympathetic component that innervates the parotid gland. Preganglionic parasympathetic neurons are located in the inferior salivatory nucleus of the medulla. They project through the tympanic and lesser petrosal nerves to the otic ganglion. Postganglionic fibers from the otic ganglion project to the parotid gland through the auriculotemporal nerve (CN V-3).

B. **CLINICAL CORRELATION.** Lesions cause the following conditions:
   1. **Loss of the gag (pharyngeal) reflex** (interruption of the afferent limb).
   2. **Hypersensitive carotid sinus reflex** (syncope).
   3. **Loss of general sensation** in the **pharynx, tonsils, fauces,** and **back of the tongue.**
   4. **Loss of taste** from the posterior one-third of the tongue.
   5. **Glossopharyngeal neuralgia,** which is characterized by severe stabbing pain in the root of the tongue.

X THE VAGAL NERVE (CN X) is a GSA, GVA, SVA, SVE, and GVE nerve (see Figure 11-7).

A. **GENERAL CHARACTERISTICS.** The vagal nerve **mediates phonation, swallowing** (with CN IX, CN XI, and CN XII), elevation of the palate, taste, and cutaneous sensation from the ear. **It innervates the viscera** of the **neck, thorax,** and **abdomen.**

   1. **Anatomy.** The vagal nerve is the nerve of pharyngeal (branchial) arches 4 and 6. Pharyngeal arch 5 is either absent or rudimentary. It exits the brain stem (medulla) from the postolivary sulcus. It exits the skull through the jugular foramen with CN IX and CN XI.

   2. The GSA **component** innervates the infratentorial dura, external ear, external auditory meatus, and tympanic membrane. It has cell bodies in the superior (jugular) ganglion, and it projects its central processes to the spinal tract and nucleus of trigeminal nerve.

   3. The GVA **component** innervates the mucous membranes of the pharynx, larynx, esophagus, trachea, and thoracic and abdominal viscera (to the left colic flexure). It has cell bodies in the inferior (nodose) ganglion. It projects its central processes to the solitary tract and nucleus.

   4. The SVA **component** innervates the taste buds in the epiglottic region. It has cell bodies in the inferior (nodose) ganglion. It projects its central processes to the solitary tract and nucleus. (For a discussion of the central pathway, see VII.A.4.d.)

   5. The SVE **component** innervates the pharyngeal (brachial) arch muscles of the larynx and pharynx, the striated muscle of the upper esophagus, the muscle of the uvula, and the levator veli palatini and palatoglossus muscles. It receives SVE input from the cranial division of the spinal accessory nerve (CN XI). It arises from the nucleus ambiguus in the lateral medulla. The SVE component provides the efferent limb of the gag reflex.

   6. The GVE **component** innervates the viscera of the neck and the thoracic (heart) and abdominal cavities as far as the left colic flexure. Preganglionic parasympathetic neurons that are located in the dorsal motor nucleus of the medulla project to the terminal (intramural) ganglia of the visceral organs.

B. CLINICAL CORRELATION. LESIONS and **reflexes** cause the following conditions:

1. **Ipsilateral paralysis** of the soft palate, pharynx, and larynx that leads to dysphonia (hoarseness), dyspnea, dysarthria, and dysphagia.
2. **Loss of the gag (palatal) reflex** (efferent limb).
3. **Anesthesia of the pharynx and larynx** that leads to unilateral loss of the cough reflex.
4. **Aortic aneurysms and tumors** of the neck and thorax that frequently compress the vagal nerve and can lead to cough, dyspnea, dysphagia, hoarseness, and chest/back pain.
5. **Complete laryngeal paralysis,** which can be rapidly fatal if it is bilateral (asphyxia).
6. **Parasympathetic (vegetative) disturbances,** including bradycardia (irritative lesion), tachycardia (destructive lesion), and dilation of the stomach.
7. The **oculocardiac reflex,** in which pressure on the eye slows the heart rate (afferent limb of CN V-1 and efferent limb of CN X).
8. The **carotid sinus reflex,** in which pressure on the carotid sinus slows the heart rate (bradycardia; efferent limb of CN X).

XI · THE ACCESSORY NERVE (CN XI), or spinal accessory nerve, is an SVE nerve (Figure 11-8).

A. GENERAL CHARACTERISTICS. The accessory nerve **mediates head and shoulder movement** and innervates the **laryngeal muscles.** It has the following divisions:

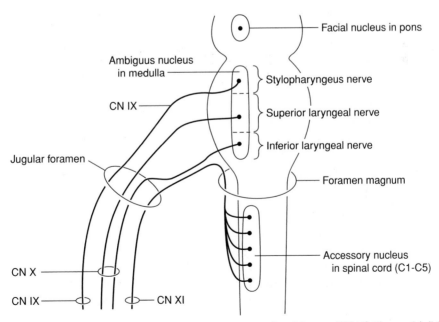

● **Figure 11-8** The cranial and spinal divisions of the accessory nerve [cranial nerve (*CN*) XI]. The cranial division hitch-hikes a ride with the accessory nerve, then joins the vagal nerve to become the inferior (recurrent) laryngeal nerve. The recurrent laryngeal nerve innervates the intrinsic muscles of the larynx, except for the cricothyroid muscle. The spinal division innervates the trapezoid and sternocleidomastoid muscles. Three nerves pass through the jugular foramen (glomus jugulare tumor). *CN*, cranial nerve.

1. The **cranial division (accessory portion)**, which arises from the nucleus ambiguus of the medulla. It exits the medulla from the postolivary sulcus and joins the vagal nerve (CN X). It exits the skull through the jugular foramen with CN IX and CN X. It **innervates** the **intrinsic muscles** of the **larynx** through the inferior (recurrent) laryngeal nerve, with the exception of the cricothyroid muscle.
2. The **spinal division (spinal portion)**, which arises from the ventral horn of cervical segments C1 through C6. The spinal roots exit the spinal cord laterally between the ventral and dorsal spinal roots, ascend through the foramen magnum, and exit the skull through the jugular foramen. It **innervates** the **sternocleidomastoid muscle** and the **trapezius muscle**.

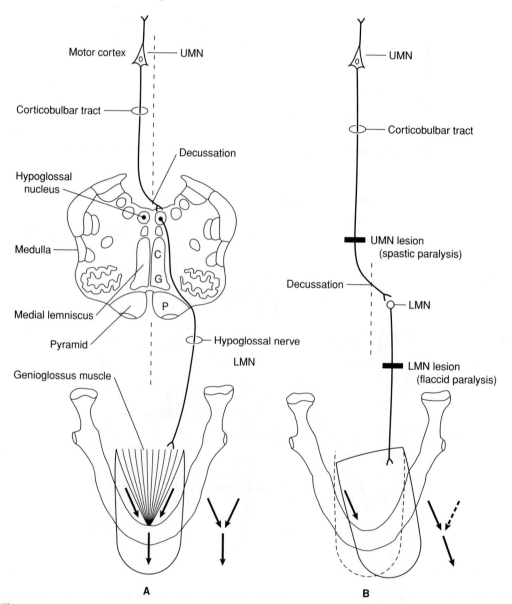

● **Figure 11-9** Motor innervation of the tongue. Corticonuclear fibers project predominantly to the contralateral hypoglossal nucleus. An upper motor neuron (*UMN*) lesion causes deviation of the protruded tongue to the weak (contralateral) side. A lower motor neuron (*LMN*) lesion causes deviation of the protruded tongue to the weak (ipsilateral) side. **(A)** Normal tongue. **(B)** Tongue with UMN and LMN lesions. (Modified from WE DeMyer, *Technique of the neurological examination: a programmed text,* 4th ed. New York: McGraw-Hill, 1994:195, with permission.)

B. **CLINICAL CORRELATION.** Lesions cause the following conditions:
1. **Paralysis of the sternocleidomastoid muscle** that results in difficulty in turning the head to the contralateral side.
2. **Paralysis of the trapezius muscle** that results in shoulder droop and inability to shrug the shoulder.
3. **Paralysis and anesthesia of the larynx** if the cranial root is involved.

XII **THE HYPOGLOSSAL NERVE (CN XII)** is a GSE nerve (Figure 11-9).

A. **GENERAL CHARACTERISTICS.** The hypoglossal nerve **mediates tongue movement.** It arises from the hypoglossal nucleus of the medulla and exits the medulla in the pre-olivary sulcus. It exits the skull through the hypoglossal canal, and it **innervates** the **intrinsic and extrinsic muscles** of the **tongue.** Extrinsic muscles are the genioglossus, styloglossus, and hyoglossus.

B. **CLINICAL CORRELATION**
1. Transection results in hemiparalysis of the tongue.
2. **Protrusion** causes the tongue to point toward the lesioned (weak) side because of the unopposed action of the opposite genioglossus muscle (Figure 11-10).

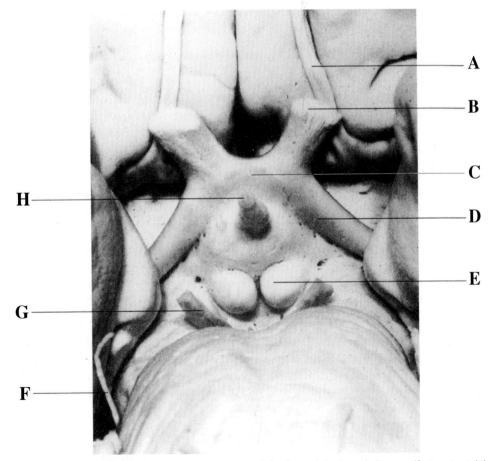

● **Figure 11-10** The basis cerebri showing cranial nerves and the floor of the hypothalamus: olfactory tract *(A)*; optic nerve *(B)*; optic chiasm *(C)*; optic tract *(D)*; mamillary body *(E)*; trochlear nerve *(F)*; oculomotor nerve *(G)*; infundibulum *(H)*. (Reprinted from JD Fix, *BRS neuroanatomy*, 3rd ed. Baltimore: Williams & Wilkins, 1996:293, with permission.)

Chapter **12**

Trigeminal System

 Key Concepts

1) Cranial nerve (CN) V-1 is the afferent limb of the corneal reflex.
2) CN V-1, V-2, III, IV, and VI and the postganglionic sympathetic fibers are all found in the cavernous sinus.

I **INTRODUCTION** The trigeminal system provides **sensory innervation to the face, oral cavity, and supratentorial dura** through general somatic afferent (GSA) fibers. It also **innervates the muscles of mastication** through special visceral efferent (SVE) fibers.

II **THE TRIGEMINAL GANGLION** (semilunar or gasserian) contains pseudounipolar ganglion cells. It has three divisions:

A. The **ophthalmic nerve [cranial nerve (CN) V-1]** lies in the wall of the cavernous sinus. It enters the orbit through the superior orbital fissure and innervates the forehead, dorsum of the nose, upper eyelid, orbit (cornea and conjunctiva), and cranial dura. The ophthalmic nerve mediates the afferent limb of the corneal reflex.

B. The **maxillary nerve (CN V-2)** lies in the wall of the cavernous sinus and innervates the upper lip and cheek, lower eyelid, anterior portion of the temple, oral mucosa of the upper mouth, nose, pharynx, gums, teeth and palate of the upper jaw, and cranial dura. It exits the skull through the foramen rotundum.

C. The **mandibular nerve (CN V-3)** exits the skull through the foramen ovale. Its **sensory (GSA) component** innervates the lower lip and chin, posterior portion of the temple, external auditory meatus, and tympanic membrane, external ear, teeth of the lower jaw, oral mucosa of the cheeks and floor of the mouth, anterior two-thirds of the tongue, temporomandibular joint, and cranial dura.

D. The **motor (SVE) component** of CN V accompanies the mandibular nerve (CN V-3) through the foramen ovale. It innervates the muscles of mastication, mylohyoid, anterior belly of the digastric, and tensores tympani and veli palatini. It innervates the muscles that move the jaw, the lateral and medial pterygoids (Figure 12-1).

III **TRIGEMINOTHALAMIC PATHWAYS** (Figure 12-2)

A. The **ventral trigeminothalamic tract** mediates pain and temperature sensation from the face and oral cavity.

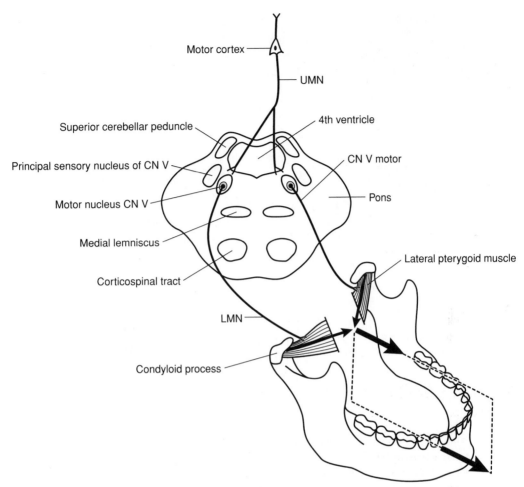

● **Figure 12-1** Function and innervation of the lateral pterygoid muscles (LPMs). The LPM receives its innervation from the motor nucleus of the trigeminal nerve found in the rostral pons. Bilateral innervation of the LPMs results in protrusion of the tip of the mandible in the midline. The LPMs also open the jaw. Denervation of one LPM results in deviation of the mandible to the ipsilateral or weak side. The trigeminal motor nucleus receives bilateral corticonuclear input. *CN*, cranial nerve; *LMN*, lower motor neuron; *UMN*, upper motor neuron. (Modified from WE DeMyer, *Technique of the neurological examination: A programmed text*, 4th ed. New York: McGraw-Hill, 1994:174, with permission.)

    1. **First-order neurons** are located in the trigeminal (gasserian) ganglion. They give rise to axons that descend in the spinal tract of trigeminal nerve and synapse with second-order neurons in the spinal nucleus of trigeminal nerve.

    2. **Second-order neurons** are located in the spinal trigeminal nucleus. They give rise to decussating axons that terminate in the contralateral ventral posteromedial (VPM) nucleus of the thalamus.

    3. **Third-order neurons** are located in the VPM nucleus of the thalamus. They project through the posterior limb of the internal capsule to the face area of the somatosensory cortex (Brodmann's areas 3, 1, and 2).

  B. The **dorsal trigeminothalamic tract** mediates tactile discrimination and pressure sensation from the face and oral cavity. It receives input from Meissner's and Pacinian corpuscles.

    1. **First-order neurons** are located in the trigeminal (gasserian) ganglion. They synapse in the principal sensory nucleus of CN V.

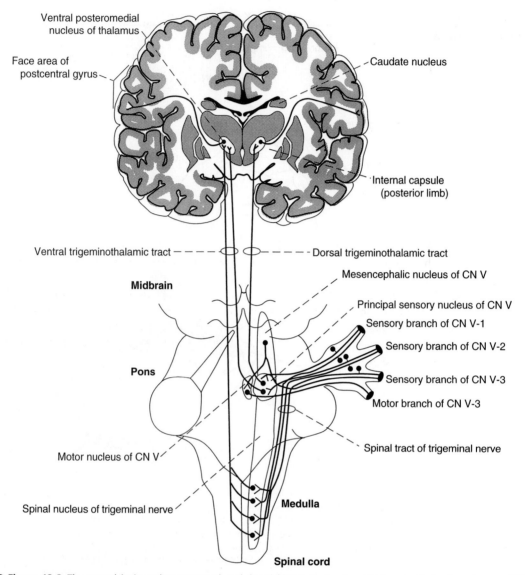

● Figure 12-2 The ventral (pain and temperature) and dorsal (discriminative touch) trigeminothalamic pathways. *CN*, cranial nerve.

2. **Second-order neurons** are located in the principal sensory nucleus of CN V. They project to the ipsilateral VPM nucleus of the thalamus.
3. **Third-order neurons** are located in the VPM nucleus of the thalamus. They project through the posterior limb of the internal capsule to the face area of the somatosensory cortex (Brodmann's areas 3, 1, and 2).

IV TRIGEMINAL REFLEXES

A. **INTRODUCTION** (Table 12-1)
   1. The **corneal reflex** is a consensual disynaptic reflex.
   2. The **jaw jerk reflex** is a monosynaptic myotactic reflex (Figure 12-3).

TABLE 12-1	THE TRIGEMINAL REFLEXES	
Reflex	**Afferent Limb**	**Efferent Limb**
Corneal reflex	Ophthalmic nerve (CN V-1)	Facial nerve (CN VII)
Jaw jerk	Mandibular nerve (CN V-3)[a]	Mandibular nerve (CN V-3)
Tearing (lacrimal) reflex	Ophthalmic nerve (CN V-1)	Facial nerve (CN VII)
Oculocardiac reflex	Ophthalmic nerve (CN V-1)	Vagal nerve (CN X)

CN, cranial nerve.
[a]The cell bodies are found in the mesencephalic nucleus of CN V.

3. The **tearing (lacrimal) reflex** occurs as a result of corneal or conjunctival irritation.
4. The **oculocardiac reflex** occurs when pressure on the globe results in **bradycardia**.

B. CLINICAL CORRELATION. Trigeminal Neuralgia (tic douloureux) is characterized by recurrent paroxysms of sharp, stabbing pain in one or more branches of the trigeminal nerve on one side of the face. It usually occurs in people older than 50 years, and it is more common in women than in men. **Carbamazepine** is the drug of choice for idiopathic trigeminal neuralgia.

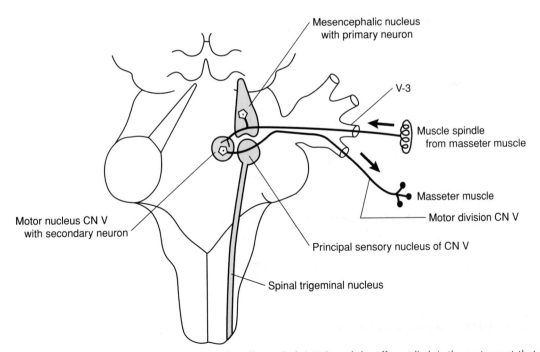

● **Figure 12-3** The jaw jerk (masseter) reflex. The afferent limb is V-3, and the efferent limb is the motor root that accompanies V-3. First-order sensory neurons are located in the mesencephalic nucleus. The jaw jerk reflex, like all muscle stretch reflexes, is a monosynaptic myotactic reflex. Hyperreflexia indicates an upper motor neuron lesion. *CN*, cranial nerve.

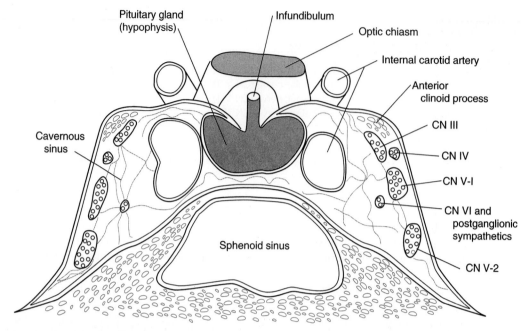

● **Figure 12-4** The contents of the cavernous sinus. The wall of the cavernous sinus contains the ophthalmic cranial nerve (*CN*) V-1 and maxillary (CN V-2) divisions of the trigeminal nerve (CN V) and the trochlear (CN IV) and oculomotor (CN III) nerves. The siphon of the internal carotid artery and the abducent nerve (CN VI), along with postganglionic sympathetic fibers, lies within the cavernous sinus.

 THE CAVERNOUS SINUS (Figure 12-4) contains the following structures:

    A. INTERNAL CAROTID ARTERY (siphon)

    B. CN III, IV, V-1, V-2, and VI

    C. POSTGANGLIONIC SYMPATHETIC FIBERS en route to the orbit

---

 Case Study

A 50-year-old woman complains of sudden onset of pain over the left side of her lower face, with the attacks consisting of brief shocks of pain that last only a few seconds at a time. Between episodes, she has no pain. Usually, the attacks are triggered by brushing her teeth, and they extend from her ear to her chin. What is the most likely diagnosis?

Relevant Physical Exam Findings

• Neurologic exam was normal to motor, sensory, and reflex testing. Magnetic resonance imaging findings were normal as well.

Diagnosis

• Trigeminal neuralgia (tic douloureux)

Chapter 13

Auditory System

 Key Concepts

1) Figure 13-1 shows an important overview of the auditory pathway.
2) What are the causes of conduction and sensorineural deafness?
3) Describe the Weber and Rinne tuning fork tests.
4) Remember that the auditory nerve and the organ of Corti are derived from the otic placode.

① INTRODUCTION The auditory system is an exteroceptive special somatic afferent system that can detect sound frequencies from 20 Hz to 20,000 Hz. It is derived from the **otic vesicle,** which is a derivative of the **otic placode,** a thickening of the **surface ectoderm.**

② THE AUDITORY PATHWAY (Figure 13-1) consists of the following structures:

A. The **hair cells of the organ of Corti** are innervated by the peripheral processes of bipolar cells of the spiral ganglion. They are stimulated by vibrations of the basilar membrane.
   1. **Inner hair cells (IHCs)** are the chief sensory elements; they synapse with dendrites of myelinated neurons whose axons make up 90% of the cochlear nerve.
   2. **Outer hair cells (OHCs)** synapse with dendrites of unmyelinated neurons whose axons make up 10% of the cochlear nerve. The OHCs reduce the threshold of the IHCs.

B. The **bipolar cells of the spiral (cochlear) ganglion** project peripherally to the hair cells of the organ of Corti. They project centrally as the cochlear nerve to the cochlear nuclei.

C. The **cochlear nerve [cranial nerve (CN) VIII]** extends from the spiral ganglion to the cerebellopontine angle, where it enters the brain stem.

D. The **cochlear nuclei** receive input from the cochlear nerve. They project contralaterally to the superior olivary nucleus and lateral lemniscus.

E. The **superior olivary nucleus,** which plays a role in sound localization, receives bilateral input from the cochlear nuclei. It projects to the lateral lemniscus.

F. The **trapezoid body** is located in the pons. It contains decussating fibers from the ventral cochlear nuclei.

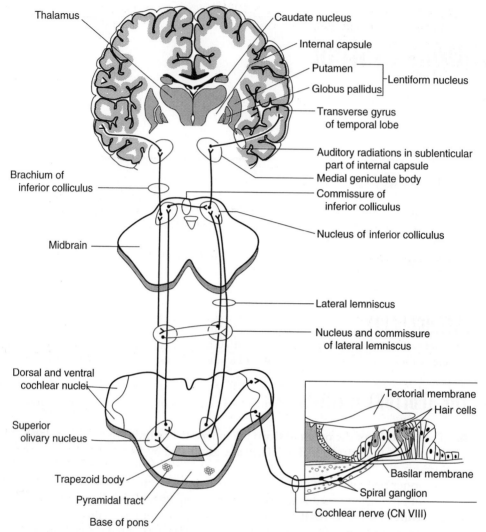

● **Figure 13-1** Peripheral and central connections of the auditory system. This system arises from the hair cells of the organ of Corti and terminates in the transverse temporal gyri of Heschl of the superior temporal gyrus. It is character-ized by the bilaterality of projections and the tonotopic localization of pitch at all levels. For example, high pitch (20,000 Hz) is localized at the base of the cochlea and in the posteromedial part of the transverse temporal gyri. *CN,* cranial nerve.

G. The **lateral lemniscus** receives input from the contralateral cochlear nuclei and superior olivary nuclei.

H. The **nucleus of inferior colliculus** receives input from the lateral lemniscus. It projects through the brachium of the inferior colliculus to the medial geniculate body.

I. The **medial geniculate body** receives input from the nucleus of the inferior colliculus. It projects through the internal capsule as the auditory radiation to the primary auditory cortex, the transverse temporal gyri of Heschl.

J. The **transverse temporal gyri of Heschl** contain the primary auditory cortex (Brodmann's areas 41 and 42). The gyri are located in the depths of the lateral sulcus.

III HEARING DEFECTS

A. CONDUCTION DEAFNESS is caused by interruption of the passage of sound waves through the external or middle ear. It may be caused by **obstruction** (e.g., wax), **otosclerosis**, or **otitis media** and is often reversible.

B. NERVE DEAFNESS (**sensorineural**, or **perceptive, deafness**) is typically permanent and is caused by disease of the cochlea, cochlear nerve (acoustic neuroma), or central auditory connections. It is usually caused by **presbycusis** that results from degenerative disease of the organ of Corti in the first few millimeters of the basal coil of the cochlea (high-frequency loss of 4,000 to 8,000 Hz).

IV AUDITORY TESTS

A. TUNING FORK TESTS (Table 13-1)
  1. Weber's test is performed by placing a vibrating tuning fork on the vertex of the skull. Normally, a patient hears equally on both sides.
    a. A patient who has **unilateral conduction deafness** hears the vibration more loudly in the affected ear.
    b. A patient who has **unilateral partial nerve deafness** hears the vibration more loudly in the normal ear.
  2. The **Rinne test** compares air and bone conduction. It is performed by placing a vibrating tuning fork on the mastoid process until the vibration is no longer heard; then the fork is held in front of the ear. Normally, a patient hears the vibration in the air after bone conduction is gone. Note that a **positive Rinne test** means that sound conduction is normal [air conduction (AC) is greater than bone conduction (BC)], whereas a **negative Rinne test** indicates conduction loss, with BC greater than AC (Table 13-1).
    a. A patient who has **unilateral conduction deafness** does not hear the vibration in the air after bone conduction is gone.
    b. A patient who has **unilateral partial nerve deafness** hears the vibration in the air after bone conduction is gone.

TABLE 13-1	TUNING FORK TEST RESULTS	
Otologic Finding	**Weber Test**	**Rinne Test**
Conduction deafness (left ear)	Lateralizes to left ear	BC >AC on left AC >BC on right
Conduction deafness (right ear)	Lateralizes to right ear	BC >AC on right AC >BC on left
Nerve deafness (left ear)	Lateralizes to right ear	AC >BC both ears
Nerve deafness (right ear)	Lateralizes to left ear	AC >BC both ears
Normal ears	No lateralization	AC >BC both ears

AC, air conduction; BC, bone conduction.

B. **BRAIN STEM AUDITORY EVOKED POTENTIALS (BAEPS)**
   1. **Testing method.** Clicks are presented to one ear, then to the other. Scalp electrodes and a computer generate a series of seven waves. The waves are associated with specific areas of the auditory pathway.
   2. **Diagnostic value.** This method is valuable for diagnosing brain stem lesions (**multiple sclerosis**) and posterior fossa tumors (**acoustic neuromas**). It is also useful for assessing hearing in infants. Approximately 50% of patients with multiple sclerosis have abnormal BAEPs.

Case Study

A 45-year-old woman presents with a 10-year history of auditory decline in her left ear. The problem began after her first pregnancy. There is no history of otologic infection or trauma. What is the most likely diagnosis?

Relevant Physical Exam Findings

- The external auditory meatus and tympanic membrane were benign bilaterally.
- The Weber test lateralized to the left side at 512 Hz, and the Rinne test was negative at 512 Hz on the left and was positive on the right.

Diagnosis

- Otosclerosis

Chapter 14

Vestibular System

 Key Concepts

1) This chapter describes the two types of vestibular nystagmus: postrotational and caloric (COWS acronym).
2) Vestibuloocular reflexes in the unconscious patient are also discussed (see Figure 14-3).

I **INTRODUCTION** Like the auditory system, the vestibular system is derived from the otic vesicle. The otic vesicle is a derivative of the **otic placode**, which is a thickening of the **surface ectoderm**. This system maintains **posture** and **equilibrium** and coordinates **head and eye movements.**

II **THE LABYRINTH**

A. KINETIC LABYRINTH
   1. **Three semicircular ducts** lie within the three semicircular canals (i.e., superior, lateral, and posterior).
   2. These ducts **respond to angular acceleration and deceleration of the head.**
      a. They contain **hair cells** in the crista ampullaris. The hair cells **respond to endolymph flow.**
      b. Endolymph flow toward the ampulla (ampullopetal) or utricle (utriculopetal) is a stronger stimulus than is endolymph flow in the opposite direction.

B. STATIC LABYRINTH
   1. The **utricle** and **saccule** respond to the position of the head with respect to **linear acceleration** and the pull of **gravity.**
   2. The utricle and saccule contain **hair cells** whose cilia are embedded in the otolithic membrane. When hair cells are bent toward the longest cilium (kinocilium), the frequency of sensory discharge increases.

III **THE VESTIBULAR PATHWAYS** (Figures 14-1 and 14-2) consist of the following structures:

A. HAIR CELLS OF THE SEMICIRCULAR DUCTS, SACCULE, AND UTRICLE are innervated by peripheral processes of **bipolar cells** of the vestibular ganglion.

B. The **vestibular ganglion** is located in the fundus of the internal auditory meatus.
   1. Bipolar neurons project through their peripheral processes to the hair cells.

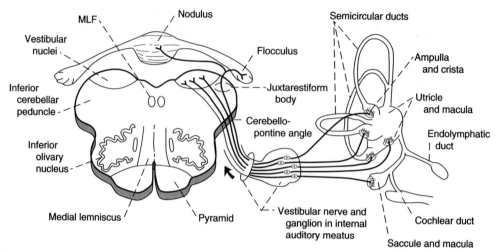

● **Figure 14-1** Peripheral connections of the vestibular system. The hair cells of the cristae ampullares and the maculae of the utricle and saccule project through the vestibular nerve to the vestibular nuclei of the medulla and pons and the flocculonodular lobe of the cerebellum (vestibulocerebellum). *MLF*, medial longitudinal fasciculus.

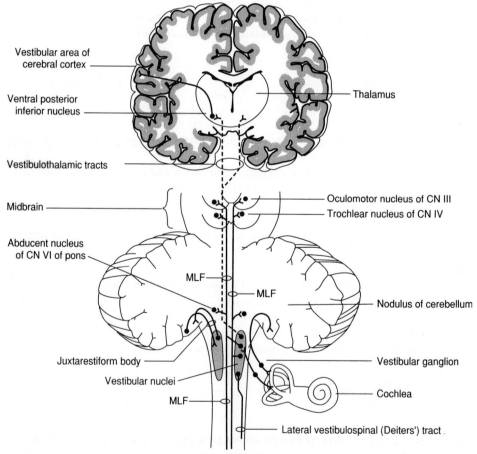

● **Figure 14-2** The major central connections of the vestibular system. Vestibular nuclei project through the ascending medial longitudinal fasciculi (*MLF*) to the ocular motor nuclei and subserve vestibuloocular reflexes. Vestibular nuclei also project through the descending MLF and lateral vestibulospinal tracts to the ventral horn motor neurons of the spinal cord and mediate postural reflexes. *CN*, cranial nerve.

2. Bipolar neurons project their central processes as the vestibular nerve [cranial nerve (CN) VIII] to the vestibular nuclei and to the flocculonodular lobe of the cerebellum.

C. VESTIBULAR NUCLEI

1. **These nuclei receive input from**
   a. The semicircular ducts, saccule, and utricle.
   b. The flocculonodular lobe of the cerebellum.
2. **The nuclei project fibers to**
   a. The flocculonodular lobe of the cerebellum.
   b. CN III, IV, and VI through the medial longitudinal fasciculus (MLF).
   c. The spinal cord through the lateral vestibulospinal tract.
   d. The ventral posteroinferior and posterolateral nuclei of the thalamus, both of which project to the postcentral gyrus.

 IV VESTIBULOOCULAR REFLEXES are mediated by the vestibular nuclei, MLF, ocular motor nuclei, and CN III, IV, and VI.

A. VESTIBULAR (HORIZONTAL) NYSTAGMUS

1. The **fast phase** of nystagmus is in the **direction of rotation**.
2. The **slow phase** of nystagmus is in the **opposite direction**.

B. POSTROTATORY (HORIZONTAL) NYSTAGMUS

1. The **fast phase** of nystagmus is in the **opposite direction of rotation**.
2. The **slow phase** of nystagmus is in the **direction of rotation**.
3. The patient past-points and falls in the direction of previous rotation.

C. CALORIC NYSTAGMUS (STIMULATION OF HORIZONTAL DUCTS) in normal subjects

1. **Cold water irrigation** of the external auditory meatus results in nystagmus to the opposite side.
2. **Warm water irrigation** of the external auditory meatus results in nystagmus to the same side.
3. **Remember the mnemonic COWS:** cold, opposite, warm, same.

D. Test results in **unconscious subjects** (Figure 14-3)

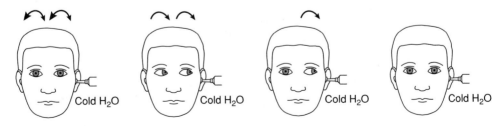

Normal conscious subject   Brain stem intact   MLF (bilateral) lesion   Low brain stem lesion

● **Figure 14-3** Cold caloric responses in the unconscious patient. When the brain stem is intact, the eyes deviate toward the irrigated side; with bilateral transection of the medial longitudinal fasciculi (*MLF*), the eye deviates to the abducted side. Destruction of the caudal brain stem results in no deviation of the eyes. *Double-headed arrows* indicate nystagmus; *single-headed arrows* indicate deviation of the eyes to one side.

1. No nystagmus is seen in normal conscious subjects.
2. When the brain stem is intact, there is deviation of the eyes to the side of the cold irrigation in unconscious subjects.
3. With bilateral MLF transaction in unconscious subjects, there is deviation of the abducting eye to the side of the cold irrigation.
4. With lower brain stem damage to the vestibular nuclei, there is no deviation of the eyes in unconscious subjects.

 # Case Study

A 60-year-old woman came to the clinic with complaints of progressive hearing loss, facial weakness, and headaches on the right side. She also said that she had become more unsteady in walking, with weakness and numbness of the right side of the face. No nausea or vomiting was noted. What is the most likely diagnosis?

Relevant Physical Exam Findings

- Reduced pain and touch sensation in right face
- Right facial weakness
- Absent right corneal reflex
- Hearing loss on right side
- No response to caloric test stimulation on right side
- Bilateral papilledema

Diagnosis

- Acoustic neuroma

Chapter 15

Visual System

 Key Concepts

1) Know the lesions of the visual system.
2) How are quadrantanopias created?
3) There are two major lesions of the optic chiasm. Know them!
4) What is Meyer's loop?

I **INTRODUCTION** The visual system is served by the optic nerve, which is a special somatic afferent nerve.

II **THE VISUAL PATHWAY** (Figure 15-1) includes the following structures:

A. GANGLION CELLS OF THE RETINA form the optic nerve [cranial nerve (CN) II]. They project from the nasal hemiretina to the contralateral lateral geniculate body and from the temporal hemiretina to the ipsilateral lateral geniculate body.

B. The **optic nerve** projects from the lamina cribrosa of the scleral canal, through the optic canal, to the optic chiasm (Figure 15-2).
   1. Transection causes ipsilateral blindness, with no direct pupillary light reflex.
   2. The section of the optic nerve at the optic chiasm transects all fibers from the ipsilateral retina and fibers from the contralateral inferior nasal quadrant that loop into the optic nerve. This **lesion** causes ipsilateral blindness and a contralateral upper temporal quadrant defect (**junction scotoma**).

C. The **optic chiasm** contains decussating fibers from the two nasal hemiretinas. It contains noncrossing fibers from the two temporal hemiretinas and projects fibers to the suprachiasmatic nucleus of the hypothalamus.
   1. Midsagittal transection or pressure (often from a pituitary tumor) causes bitemporal hemianopia.
   2. Bilateral lateral compression causes binasal hemianopia (calcified internal carotid arteries).

D. The **optic tract** contains fibers from the ipsilateral temporal hemiretina and the contralateral nasal hemiretina. It projects to the ipsilateral lateral geniculate body, pretectal nuclei, and superior colliculus. Transection causes contralateral hemianopia.

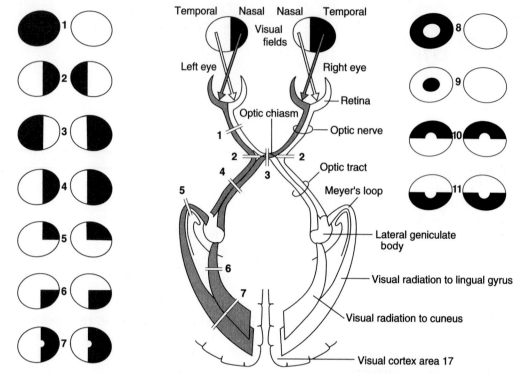

● Figure 15-1 The visual pathway from the retina to the visual cortex showing visual field defects. *(1)* Ipsilateral blindness. *(2)* Binasal hemianopia. *(3)* Bitemporal hemianopia. *(4)* Right hemianopia. *(5)* Right upper quadrantanopia. *(6)* Right lower quadrantanopia. *(7)* Right hemianopia with macular sparing. *(8)* Left constricted field as a result of end-stage glaucoma. Bilateral constricted fields may be seen in hysteria. *(9)* Left central scotoma as seen in optic (retrobulbar) neuritis in multiple sclerosis. *(10)* Upper altitudinal hemianopia as a result of bilateral destruction of the lingual gyri. *(11)* Lower altitudinal hemianopia as a result of bilateral destruction of the cunei.

E. The **lateral geniculate body** is a six-layered nucleus. Layers 1, 4, and 6 receive crossed fibers; layers 2, 3, and 5 receive uncrossed fibers. The lateral geniculate body receives input from layer VI of the striate cortex (Brodmann's area 17). It also receives fibers from the ipsilateral temporal hemiretina and the contralateral nasal hemiretina. It projects through the geniculocalcarine tract to layer IV of the primary visual cortex (Brodmann's area 17).

F. The **geniculocalcarine tract (visual radiation)** projects through two divisions to the visual cortex.
1. The **upper division** (Figure 15-3) projects to the upper bank of the calcarine sulcus, the cuneus. It contains input from the superior retinal quadrants, which represent the inferior visual-field quadrants.
   a. **Transection** causes a contralateral lower quadrantanopia.
   b. **Lesions** that involve both cunei cause a lower altitudinal hemianopia (altitudinopia).
2. The **lower division** (see Figure 15-3) loops from the lateral geniculate body anteriorly (Meyer's loop), then posteriorly, to terminate in the lower bank of the calcarine sulcus, the lingual gyrus. It contains input from the inferior retinal quadrants, which represent the superior visual field quadrants.
   a. **Transection** causes a **contralateral upper quadrantanopia** ("pie in the sky").
   b. **Transection** of both lingual gyri causes an **upper altitudinal hemianopia (altitudinopia).**

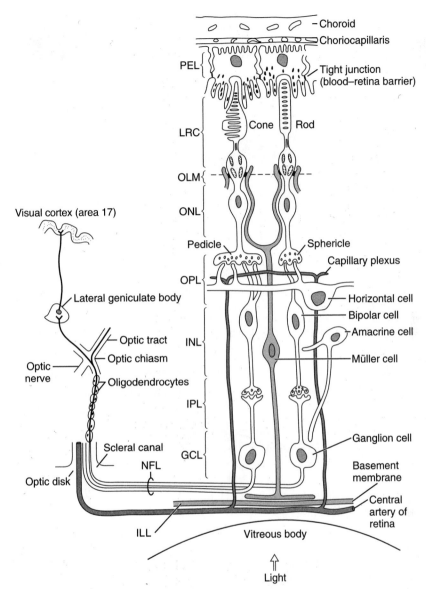

● **Figure 15-2** Histology of the retina. The retina has 10 layers: (1) pigment epithelium layer *(PEL)*, (2) layer of rods and cones *(LRC)*, (3) outer limiting membrane *(OLM)*, (4) outer nuclear layer *(ONL)*, (5) outer plexiform layer *(OPL)*, (6) inner nuclear layer *(INL)*, (7) inner plexiform layer *(IPL)*, (8) ganglion cell layer *(GCL)*, (9) nerve fiber layer *(NFL)*, and (10) inner limiting layer *(ILL)*. The tight junctions binding the pigment epithelial cells make up the blood–retina barrier. Retinal detachment usually occurs between the pigment layer and the layer of rods and cones. The central artery of the retina perfuses the retina to the outer plexiform layer, and the choriocapillaris supplies the outer five layers of the retina. The Müller cells are radial glial cells that have support function. Myelin of the central nervous system (CNS) is produced by oligodendrocytes, which are not normally found in the retina. (Adapted from RW Dudek, *High-yield histology*. Baltimore: Williams & Wilkins, 1997:64, with permission.)

    G. The **visual cortex (Brodmann's area 17)** is located on the banks of the calcarine fissure. **The cuneus** is the upper bank. The **lingual gyrus** is the lower bank. Lesions cause **contralateral hemianopia** with macular sparing. The visual cortex has a **retinotopic organization:**

      1. The **posterior area** receives macular input (central vision).

      2. The **intermediate area** receives paramacular input (peripheral input).

      3. The **anterior area** receives monocular input.

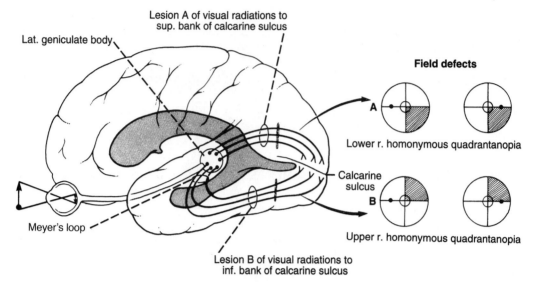

● **Figure 15-3** Relations of the left upper and left lower divisions of the geniculocalcarine tract to the lateral ventricle and calcarine sulcus. Transection of the upper division **(A)** results in right lower homonymous quadrantanopia. Transection of the lower division **(B)** results in right upper homonymous quadrantanopia. (Reprinted from JD Fix, *BRS neuroanatomy*. Baltimore: Williams & Wilkins, 1997:261, with permission.)

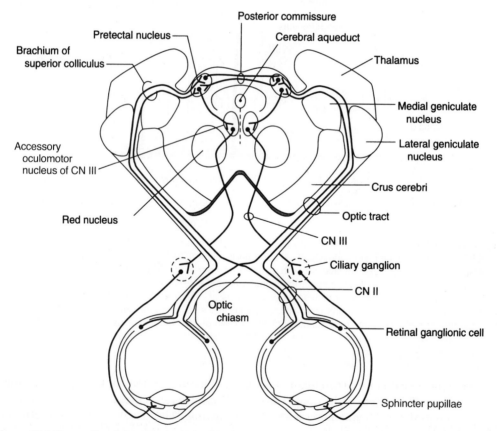

● **Figure 15-4** The pupillary light pathway. Light shined into one eye causes both pupils to constrict. The response in the stimulated eye is called the *direct pupillary light reflex*. The response in the opposite eye is called the *consensual pupillary light reflex. CN*, cranial nerve.

III **THE PUPILLARY LIGHT REFLEX PATHWAY** (Figure 15-4) has an afferent limb (CN II) and an efferent limb (CN III). It includes the following structures:

A. GANGLION CELLS OF THE RETINA, which project bilaterally to the pretectal nuclei.

B. The **pretectal nucleus of the midbrain**, which projects (through the posterior commissure) crossed and uncrossed fibers to the accessory oculomotor (Edinger-Westphal) nucleus.

C. The **accessory oculomotor** (Edinger-Westphal) **nucleus of CN III**, which gives rise to preganglionic parasympathetic fibers. These fibers exit the midbrain with CN III and synapse with postganglionic parasympathetic neurons of the ciliary ganglion.

D. The **ciliary ganglion**, which gives rise to postganglionic parasympathetic fibers. These fibers innervate the sphincter muscle of the iris.

IV **THE PUPILLARY DILATION PATHWAY** (Figure 15-5) is mediated by the sympathetic division of the autonomic nervous system. Interruption of this pathway at any level causes ipsilateral Horner's syndrome. It includes the following structures:

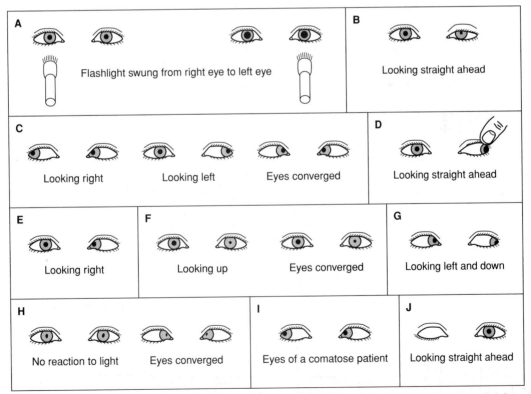

● **Figure 15-5** Ocular motor palsies and pupillary syndromes. **(A)** Relative afferent (Marcus Gunn) pupil, left eye. **(B)** Horner's syndrome, left eye. **(C)** Internuclear ophthalmoplegia, right eye. **(D)** Third-nerve palsy, left eye. **(E)** Sixth-nerve palsy, right eye. **(F)** Paralysis of upward gaze and convergence (Parinaud's syndrome). **(G)** Fourth-nerve palsy, right eye. **(H)** Argyll Robertson pupil. **(I)** Destructive lesion of the right frontal eye field. **(J)** Third-nerve palsy with ptosis, right eye.

A. The **hypothalamus**. Hypothalamic neurons of the paraventricular nucleus project directly to the ciliospinal center (T1–T2) of the intermediolateral cell column of the spinal cord.

B. The **ciliospinal center of Budge (T1–T2)** projects preganglionic sympathetic fibers through the sympathetic trunk to the superior cervical ganglion.

C. The **superior cervical ganglion** projects postganglionic sympathetic fibers through the perivascular plexus of the carotid system to the dilator muscle of the iris. Postganglionic sympathetic fibers pass through the **tympanic cavity** and **cavernous sinus** and enter the orbit through the **superior orbital fissure**.

V THE NEAR REFLEX AND ACCOMMODATION PATHWAY

A. The **cortical visual pathway** projects from the primary visual cortex (Brodmann's area 17) to the visual association cortex (Brodmann's area 19).

B. The **visual association cortex (Brodmann's area 19)** projects through the corticotectal tract to the superior colliculus and pretectal nucleus.

C. The **superior colliculus** and **pretectal nucleus** project to the **oculomotor complex** of the **midbrain**. This complex includes the following structures:
   1. The **rostral accessory oculomotor (Edinger-Westphal) nucleus**, which mediates pupillary constriction through the ciliary ganglion.
   2. The **caudal accessory oculomotor (Edinger-Westphal) nucleus**, which mediates contraction of the ciliary muscle. This contraction increases the refractive power of the lens.
   3. The **medial rectus subnucleus of CN III**, which mediates convergence.

VI CORTICAL AND SUBCORTICAL CENTERS FOR OCULAR MOTILITY

A. The **frontal eye field** is located in the posterior part of the middle frontal gyrus (Brodmann's area 8). It regulates voluntary (saccadic) eye movements.
   1. Stimulation (e.g., from an irritative lesion) causes **contralateral deviation of the eyes** (i.e., away from the lesion).
   2. Destruction causes **transient ipsilateral conjugate deviation of the eyes** (i.e., toward the lesion).

B. OCCIPITAL EYE FIELDS are located in Brodmann's areas 18 and 19 of the occipital lobes. These fields are cortical centers for involuntary (smooth) pursuit and tracking movements. **Stimulation** causes contralateral conjugate deviation of the eyes.

C. The **subcortical center for lateral conjugate gaze** is located in the abducent nucleus of the pons (Figure 15-6). Some authorities place the "center" in the paramedian pontine reticular formation.
   1. It receives input from the contralateral frontal eye field.
   2. It projects to the ipsilateral lateral rectus muscle and through the medial longitudinal fasciculus (MLF) to the contralateral medial rectus subnucleus of the oculomotor complex.

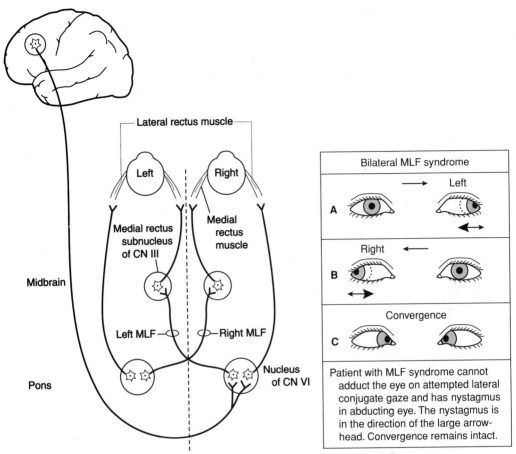

● **Figure 15-6** Connections of the pontine center for lateral conjugate gaze. Lesions of the medial longitudinal fasciculus (*MLF*) between the abducent and oculomotor nuclei result in medial rectus palsy on attempted lateral conjugate gaze and horizontal nystagmus in the abducting eye. Convergence remains intact (*inset*). A unilateral MLF lesion would affect only the ipsilateral medial rectus. *CN*, cranial nerve.

D. The **subcortical center for vertical conjugate gaze** is located in the midbrain at the level of the posterior commissure. It is called the *rostral interstitial nucleus of the MLF* and is associated with **Parinaud's syndrome** (see Figures 15-5F and 16-3A).

VII CLINICAL CORRELATION

A. In **MLF syndrome**, or **internuclear ophthalmoplegia** (see Figure 15-5), there is damage (demyelination) to the MLF between the abducent and oculomotor nuclei. It causes **medial rectus palsy on attempted lateral conjugate gaze** and monocular horizontal nystagmus in the abducting eye. (**Convergence is normal.**) This syndrome is most commonly seen in **multiple sclerosis.**

B. **ONE-AND-A-HALF SYNDROME** consists of bilateral lesions of the MLF and a unilateral lesion of the abducent nucleus. On attempted lateral conjugate gaze, the only muscle that functions is the intact lateral rectus.

C.   ARGYLL ROBERTSON PUPIL (pupillary light–near dissociation) is the absence of a miotic reaction to light, both direct and consensual, with the preservation of a miotic reaction to near stimulus (accommodation–convergence). It occurs in **syphilis** and **diabetes.**

D.   HORNER'S SYNDROME is caused by transection of the oculosympathetic pathway at any level (see IV). This syndrome consists of miosis, ptosis, apparent enophthalmos, and hemianhidrosis.

E.   RELATIVE AFFERENT (MARCUS GUNN) PUPIL results from a lesion of the optic nerve, the afferent limb of the pupillary light reflex (e.g., retrobulbar neuritis seen in multiple sclerosis). The diagnosis can be made with the swinging flashlight test (see Figure 15-5A).

F.   TRANSTENTORIAL (UNCAL) HERNIATION occurs as a result of **increased supratentorial pressure,** which is commonly caused by a brain tumor or hematoma (subdural or epidural).

    1.   The pressure cone forces the parahippocampal uncus through the tentorial incisure.

    2.   The impacted uncus forces the contralateral crus cerebri against the tentorial edge (Kernohan's notch) and puts pressure on the ipsilateral CN III and posterior cerebral artery. As a result, the following neurologic defects occur.

        a.   **Ipsilateral hemiparesis** occurs as a result of pressure on the corticospinal tract, which is located in the contralateral crus cerebri.

        b.   A **fixed and dilated pupil, ptosis,** and a **"down-and-out" eye** are caused by pressure on the ipsilateral oculomotor nerve.

        c.   **Contralateral homonymous hemianopia** is caused by compression of the posterior cerebral artery, which irrigates the visual cortex.

G.   PAPILLEDEMA (CHOKED DISK) is noninflammatory congestion of the optic disk as a result of increased intracranial pressure. It is most commonly caused by brain tumors, subdural hematoma, or hydrocephalus. It usually **does not alter visual acuity,** but it may cause bilateral **enlarged blind spots.** It is often asymmetric and is greater on the side of the supratentorial lesion.

H.   ADIE'S PUPIL is a large tonic pupil that reacts slowly to light but does react to near (light–near dissociation). It is frequently seen in women with absent knee or ankle jerks.

🔾 Case Study

A 40-year-old man comes to the clinic with a severe unilateral headache on the left side with a drooping left upper eyelid. He experienced mild head trauma 1 week ago. He does not complain of blurred or double vision. What is the most likely diagnosis?

Relevant Physical Exam Findings

- The right pupil is 4 mm and normally reactive, and the left pupil is 2 mm and normally reactive.
- The left pupil dilates poorly.
- There is 2- to 3-mm ptosis of the left upper eyelid.

Diagnosis

- Horner's syndrome.

Chapter 16

Lesions of the Brain Stem

 Key Concepts

1) The three most important lesions of the brain stem are occlusion of the anterior spinal artery (Figure 16-1), occlusion of the posterior inferior cerebellar artery (Figure 16-1), and medial longitudinal fasciculus syndrome (Figure 16-2).
2) Weber's syndrome is the most common midbrain lesion (Figure 16-3).

I LESIONS OF THE MEDULLA (Figure 16-1)

A. MEDIAL MEDULLARY SYNDROME (ANTERIOR SPINAL ARTERY SYNDROME). Affected structures and resultant deficits include
   1. The **corticospinal tract** (medullary pyramid). Lesions result in contralateral spastic hemiparesis.
   2. The **medial lemniscus.** Lesions result in contralateral loss of tactile and vibration sensation from the trunk and extremities.
   3. The **hypoglossal nucleus or intraaxial root fibers [cranial nerve (CN) XII].** Lesions result in ipsilateral flaccid hemiparalysis of the tongue. When protruded, the tongue points to the side of the lesion (i.e., the weak side). See Figure 11-9.

B. LATERAL MEDULLARY [WALLENBERG; POSTERIOR INFERIOR CEREBELLAR ARTERY (PICA)] SYNDROME is characterized by dissociated sensory loss (see I.B.6–7). Affected structures and resultant deficits include
   1. The **vestibular nuclei.** Lesions result in nystagmus, nausea, vomiting, and vertigo.
   2. The **inferior cerebellar peduncle.** Lesions result in ipsilateral cerebellar signs [e.g., dystaxia, dysmetria (past pointing), dysdiadochokinesia].
   3. The **nucleus ambiguus of CN IX, CN X, and CN XI.** Lesions result in ipsilateral laryngeal, pharyngeal, and palatal hemiparalysis [i.e., loss of the gag reflex (efferent limb), dysarthria, dysphagia, and dysphonia (hoarseness)].
   4. The **glossopharyngeal nerve roots.** Lesions result in loss of the gag reflex (afferent limb).
   5. The **vagal nerve roots.** Lesions result in the same deficits as seen in lesions involving the nucleus ambiguus (see I.B.3).
   6. The **spinothalamic tracts (spinal lemniscus).** Lesions result in contralateral loss of pain and temperature sensation from the trunk and extremities.
   7. The **spinal trigeminal nucleus and tract.** Lesions result in ipsilateral loss of pain and temperature sensation from the face (facial hemianesthesia).
   8. The **descending sympathetic tract.** Lesions result in ipsilateral Horner's syndrome (i.e., ptosis, miosis, hemianhidrosis, and apparent enophthalmos).

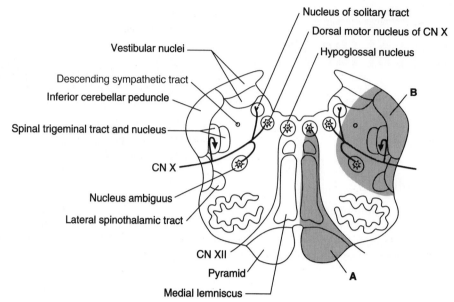

Figure 16-1 Vascular lesions of the medulla at the level of the hypoglossal nucleus of cranial nerve (*CN*) XII and the dorsal motor nucleus of CN X. *(A)* Medial medullary syndrome (anterior spinal artery). *(B)* Lateral medullary (posterior inferior cerebellar artery) syndrome.

LESIONS OF THE PONS (Figure 16-2A)

A. MEDIAL INFERIOR PONTINE SYNDROME results from occlusion of the paramedian branches of the basilar artery. Affected structures and resultant deficits include

   1. The **corticospinal tract.** Lesions result in contralateral spastic hemiparesis.

   2. The **medial lemniscus.** Lesions result in contralateral loss of tactile sensation from the trunk and extremities.

   3. The **abducent nerve roots.** Lesions result in ipsilateral lateral rectus paralysis.

B. LATERAL INFERIOR PONTINE SYNDROME (anterior inferior cerebellar artery syndrome; Figure 16-2B). Affected structures and resultant deficits include

   1. The **facial nucleus and intraaxial nerve fibers.** Lesions result in

   a. Ipsilateral facial nerve paralysis.

   b. Ipsilateral loss of taste from the anterior two-thirds of the tongue.

   c. Ipsilateral loss of lacrimation and reduced salivation.

   d. Loss of corneal and stapedial reflexes (efferent limbs).

   2. The **cochlear nuclei and intraaxial nerve fibers.** Lesions result in unilateral central deafness.

   3. The **vestibular nuclei and intraaxial nerve fibers.** Lesions result in nystagmus, nausea, vomiting, and vertigo.

   4. The **spinal nucleus and tract of trigeminal nerve.** Lesions result in ipsilateral loss of pain and temperature sensation from the face (facial hemianesthesia).

   5. The **middle and inferior cerebellar peduncles.** Lesions result in ipsilateral limb and gait dystaxia.

   6. The **spinothalamic tracts (spinal lemniscus).** Lesions result in contralateral loss of pain and temperature sensation from the trunk and extremities.

   7. The **descending sympathetic tract.** Lesions result in ipsilateral Horner's syndrome.

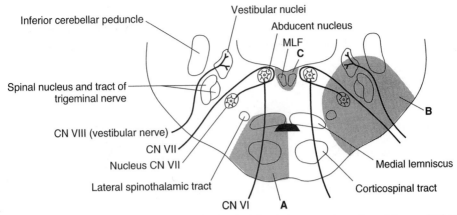

Figure 16-2 Vascular lesions of the caudal pons at the level of the abducent nucleus of cranial nerve (*CN*) VI and the facial nucleus of CN VII. *(A)* Medial inferior pontine syndrome. *(B)* Lateral inferior pontine syndrome (anterior inferior cerebellar artery syndrome). *(C)* Medial longitudinal fasciculus (*MLF*) syndrome.

C. **MEDIAL LONGITUDINAL FASCICULUS (MLF) SYNDROME (INTERNUCLEAR OPHTHALMOPLEGIA)** (Figure 16-2C) interrupts fibers from the contralateral abducent nucleus that project through the MLF to the ipsilateral medial rectus subnucleus of CN III. It causes **medial rectus palsy** on attempted lateral conjugate gaze and **nystagmus** in the abducting eye. Convergence remains intact. This syndrome is often seen in patients with **multiple sclerosis.**

D. **FACIAL COLLICULUS SYNDROME** usually results from a pontine glioma or a vascular accident. The internal genu of CN VII and the nucleus of CN VI underlie the facial colliculus.
   1. Lesions of the **internal genu** of the **facial nerve** cause
      a. Ipsilateral facial paralysis.
      b. Ipsilateral loss of the corneal reflex.
   2. Lesions of the **abducent nucleus** cause
      a. Lateral rectus paralysis.
      b. Medial (convergent) strabismus.
      c. Horizontal diplopia.

III **LESIONS OF THE MIDBRAIN** (Figure 16-3)

A. **DORSAL MIDBRAIN (PARINAUD'S) SYNDROME** (see Figure 16-3A) is often the result of a pinealoma or germinoma of the pineal region. Affected structures and resultant deficits include
   1. The **superior colliculus** and **pretectal area.** Lesions cause paralysis of upward and downward gaze, pupillary disturbances, and absence of convergence.
   2. The **cerebral aqueduct.** Compression causes noncommunicating hydrocephalus.

B. **PARAMEDIAN MIDBRAIN (BENEDIKT'S) SYNDROME** (see Figure 16-3B). Affected structures and resultant deficits include
   1. The **oculomotor nerve roots** (intraaxial fibers). Lesions cause complete ipsilateral oculomotor paralysis. Eye abduction and depression is caused by the intact lateral

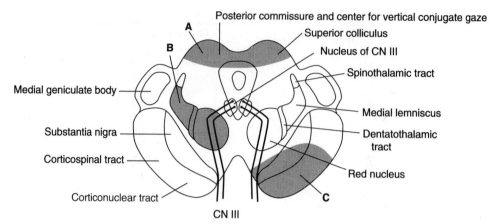

Figure 16-3 Lesions of the rostral midbrain at the level of the superior colliculus and oculomotor nucleus of cranial nerve (*CN*) III. *(A)* Dorsal midbrain (Parinaud's) syndrome. *(B)* Paramedian midbrain (Benedikt's) syndrome. *(C)* Medial midbrain (Weber's) syndrome.

rectus (CN VI) and superior oblique (CN IV) muscles. Ptosis (paralysis of the levator palpebrae superioris muscle) and fixation and dilation of the ipsilateral pupil (complete internal ophthalmoplegia) also occur.

2. The **dentatothalamic fibers.** Lesions cause contralateral cerebellar dystaxia with intention tremor.

3. The **medial lemniscus.** Lesions result in contralateral loss of tactile sensation from the trunk and extremities.

C. MEDIAL MIDBRAIN (WEBER'S) SYNDROME (see Figure 16-3C). Affected structures and resultant deficits include

1. The **oculomotor nerve roots** (intraaxial fibers). Lesions cause complete ipsilateral oculomotor paralysis. Eye abduction and depression are caused by intact lateral rectus (CN VI) and superior oblique (CN IV) muscles. Ptosis and fixation and dilation of the ipsilateral pupil also occur.

2. The **corticospinal tracts.** Lesions result in contralateral spastic hemiparesis.

3. The **corticonuclear fibers.** Lesions cause contralateral weakness of the lower face (CN VII), tongue (CN XII), and palate (CN X). The upper face division of the facial nucleus receives bilateral corticonuclear input. The uvula and pharyngeal wall are pulled toward the normal side (CN X), and the protruded tongue points to the weak side.

IV ACOUSTIC NEUROMA (SCHWANNOMA) (Figure 16-4) is a benign tumor of Schwann cells that affects the vestibulocochlear nerve (CN VIII). It accounts for 8% of all intracranial tumors. It is a posterior fossa tumor of the internal auditory meatus and cerebellopontine angle. The neuroma often compresses the facial nerve (CN VII), which accompanies CN VIII in the cerebellopontine angle and internal auditory meatus. It may impinge on the pons and affect the spinal trigeminal tract (CN V). **Schwannomas** occur twice as often in women as in men. Affected structures and resultant deficits include

A. The **cochlear nerve of CN VIII.** Damage results in tinnitus and unilateral nerve deafness.

B. The **vestibular nerve of CN VIII.** Damage results in vertigo, nystagmus, nausea, vomiting, and unsteadiness of gait.

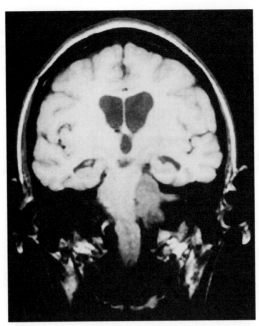

Figure 16-4 Magnetic resonance image of an acoustic neuroma. This coronal section shows dilation of the ventricles. The vestibulocochlear nerve is visible in the left internal auditory meatus. The tumor indents the lateral pons. Cranial nerve (CN) palsies include CN V, VII, and VIII. Symptoms include unilateral deafness, facial anesthesia and weakness, and an absent coronal reflex. This is a T1-weighted image.

C. The **facial nerve (CN VII)**. Damage results in facial weakness and loss of the corneal reflex (efferent limb).

D. The **spinal tract of trigeminal nerve (CN V)**. Damage results in paresthesia, anesthesia of the ipsilateral face, and loss of the corneal reflex (afferent limb).

E. NEUROFIBROMATOSIS TYPE 2. This disorder often occurs with bilateral acoustic neuromas.

V JUGULAR FORAMEN SYNDROME usually results from a posterior fossa tumor (e.g., **glomus jugulare tumor,** the most common inner ear tumor) that compresses CN IX, X, and XI. Affected structures and resultant deficits include

A. The **glossopharyngeal nerve (CN IX)**. Damage results in
   1. Ipsilateral loss of the gag reflex.
   2. Ipsilateral loss of pain, temperature, and taste in the tongue.

B. The **vagal nerve (CN X)**. Damage results in
   1. Ipsilateral paralysis of the soft palate and larynx.
   2. Ipsilateral loss of the gag reflex.

C. The **accessory nerve (CN XI)**. Damage results in
   1. Paralysis of the sternocleidomastoid muscle, which results in the inability to turn the head to the opposite side.
   2. Paralysis of the trapezius muscle, which causes shoulder droop and inability to shrug the shoulder.

VI **"LOCKED-IN" SYNDROME** is a lesion of the base of the pons as the result of infarction, trauma, tumor, or demyelination. The corticospinal and corticonuclear tracts are affected bilaterally. The oculomotor and trochlear nerves are not injured. Patients are conscious and may communicate through vertical eye movements.

VII **CENTRAL PONTINE MYELINOLYSIS** is a lesion of the base of the pons that affects the corticospinal and corticobulbar tracts. More than 75% of cases are associated with alcoholism or rapid correction of hyponatremia. Symptoms include spastic quadriparesis, pseudobulbar palsy, and mental changes. This condition may become the locked-in syndrome.

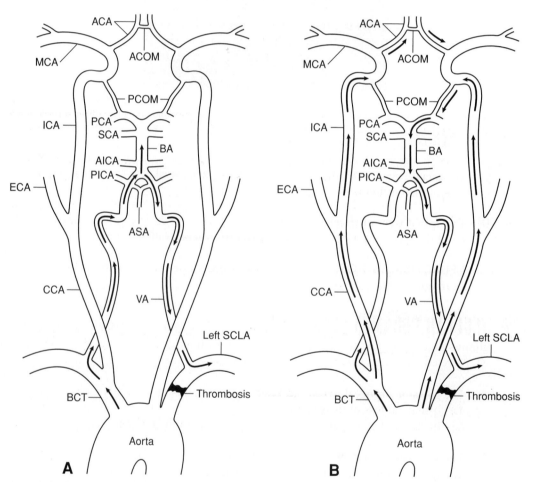

Figure 16-5 Anatomy of the subclavian steal syndrome. Thrombosis of the proximal part of the subclavian artery (left) results in retrograde blood flow through the ipsilateral vertebral artery and into the left subclavian artery. Blood can be shunted from the right vertebral artery and down the left vertebral artery **(A)**. Blood may also reach the left vertebral artery through the carotid circulation **(B)**. *ACA*, anterior cerebellar artery; *ACOM*, anterior communicating artery; *AICA*, anterior inferior cerebellar artery; *ASA*, anterior spinal artery; *BA*, basilar artery; *BCT*, brachiocephalic trunk; *CCA*, common carotid artery; *ECA*, external carotid artery; *ICA*, internal carotid artery; *MCA*, middle cerebral artery; *PCA*, posterior cerebral artery; *PCOM*, posterior communicating artery; *PICA*, posterior inferior cerebellar artery; *SCA*, superior communicating artery; *SCLA*, subclavian artery; *VA*, vertebral artery.

VIII **"TOP OF THE BASILAR" SYNDROME** results from embolic occlusion of the rostral basilar artery. Neurologic signs include optic ataxia and psychic paralysis of fixation of gaze (**Balint's syndrome**), ectopic pupils, somnolence, and cortical blindness, with or without visual anosognosia (**Anton's syndrome**).

IX **SUBCLAVIAN STEAL SYNDROME** (Figure 16-5) results from thrombosis of the left subclavian artery proximal to the vertebral artery. Blood is shunted retrograde down the left vertebral artery and into the left subclavian artery. Clinical signs include transient weakness and claudication of the left arm on exercise and vertebrobasilar insufficiency (i.e., vertigo, dizziness).

X **THE CEREBELLOPONTINE ANGLE** is the junction of the medulla, pons, and cerebellum. CN VII and VIII are found there. Five brain tumors, including a cyst, are often located in the cerebellopontine angle cistern. Remember the acronym **SAME:** schwannoma (75%), arachnoid cyst (1%), meningioma (10%), and ependymoma (1%) and epidermoid (5%). The percentages refer to cerebellopontine angle tumors.

Case Study

For several weeks, a 60-year-old hypertensive, diabetic man has experienced sudden dizziness, facial pain, double vision, and difficulty in walking. He is also having problems in swallowing and speaking. What is the most likely diagnosis?

Relevant Physical Exam Findings

- Decreased temperature and pain sense below the left T-4 level
- Horner's syndrome on the right side
- Decreased position sensation in the right fingers and toes
- Ataxia and mild weakness in the right limbs

Relevant Lab Finding

- An infarct involving the right lateral part of the lower medulla and the cerebellum seen on brain magnetic resonance image

Diagnosis

- Wallenberg's syndrome is an infarction involving the lateral or medial branches of the posterior inferior cerebellar artery.

Chapter 17

Thalamus

Key Concepts

1) Key entry and exit points into and out of the thalamus (demonstrated by Figure 17-1).
2) Anatomy of the internal capsule. (It will be on the examination.) What is the blood supply of the internal capsule (stroke)?

I **INTRODUCTION** The thalamus is the largest division of the diencephalon. It plays an important role in the integration of the sensory and motor systems.

II **MAJOR THALAMIC NUCLEI AND THEIR CONNECTIONS** (Figure 17-1)

A. The anterior nucleus receives hypothalamic input from the mamillary nucleus through the mamillothalamic tract. It projects to the cingulate gyrus and is part of the Papez circuit of emotion of the limbic system.

B. The **mediodorsal (dorsomedial) nucleus** is reciprocally connected to the prefrontal cortex. It has abundant connections with the **intralaminar nuclei**. It receives input from the amygdale, substantia nigra, and temporal neocortex. When it is destroyed, **memory loss** occurs (Wernicke-Korsakoff syndrome). The mediodorsal nucleus plays a role in the expression of affect, emotion, and behavior (limbic function).

C. The **centromedian nucleus** is the largest intralaminar nucleus. It is reciprocally connected to the motor cortex (Brodmann's area 4). The centromedian nucleus receives input from the globus pallidus. It projects to the striatum (caudate nucleus and putamen) and projects diffusely to the entire neocortex.

D. The **pulvinar** is the largest thalamic nucleus. It has reciprocal connections with the association cortex of the occipital, parietal, and posterior temporal lobes. It receives input from the lateral and medial geniculate bodies and the superior colliculus. It plays a role in the **integration of visual**, **auditory**, and **somesthetic input**. Destruction of the dominant pulvinar may result in sensory dysphasia.

E. **VENTRAL TIER NUCLEI**
    1. The **ventral anterior nucleus** receives input from the globus pallidus and substantia nigra. It projects diffusely to the prefrontal cortex, orbital cortex, and premotor cortex (Brodmann's area 6).

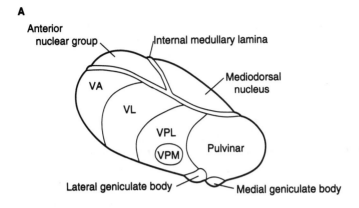

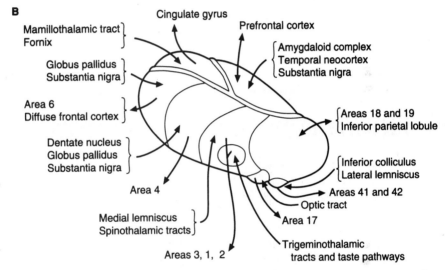

Figure 17-1 Major thalamic nuclei and their connections. **(A)** Dorsolateral aspect and major nuclei. **(B)** Major afferent and efferent connections. *VA*, ventral anterior nucleus; *VL*, ventral lateral nucleus; *VPL*, ventral posterior lateral nucleus; *VPM*, ventral posterior medial nucleus.

2. The **ventral lateral nucleus** receives input from the cerebellum (dentate nucleus), globus pallidus, and substantia nigra. It projects to the motor cortex (Brodmann's area 4) and the supplementary motor cortex (Brodmann's area 6).

3. The **ventral posterior nucleus** (ventrobasal complex) is the nucleus of termination of general somatic afferent (touch, pain, and temperature) and special visceral afferent (taste) fibers. It has two subnuclei.

    a. The **ventral posterolateral nucleus** receives the spinothalamic tracts and the medial lemniscus. It projects to the somesthetic (sensory) cortex (Brodmann's areas 3, 1, and 2).

    b. The **ventral posteromedial (VPM) nucleus** receives the trigeminothalamic tracts and projects to the somesthetic (sensory) cortex (Brodmann's areas 3, 1, and 2). The gustatory (taste) pathway originates in the solitary nucleus and projects via the central tegmental tract to the VPM and thence to the gustatory cortex of the postcentral gyrus (Brodmann's area 3b), of the frontal operculum, and of the insular cortex. The taste pathway is ipsilateral.

F.   METATHALAMUS

1.   The **lateral geniculate body** is a visual relay nucleus. It receives retinal input through the optic tract and projects to the primary visual cortex (Brodmann's area 17).

2.   The **medial geniculate body** is an auditory relay nucleus. It receives auditory input through the brachium of the inferior colliculus and projects to the primary auditory cortex (Brodmann's areas 41 and 42).

G.   The **reticular nucleus of the thalamus** surrounds the thalamus as a thin layer of γ-aminobutyric acid (GABA)-ergic neurons. It lies between the external medullary lamina and the internal capsule. It receives excitatory collateral input from corticothalamic and thalamocortical fibers. It projects inhibitory fibers to thalamic nuclei, from which it receives input. It is thought to play a role in normal electroencephalogram readings.

III   BLOOD SUPPLY   The thalamus is irrigated by three arteries (see Figure 5-1):

A.   The **posterior communicating artery.**

B.   The **posterior cerebral artery.**

C.   The **anterior choroidal artery** (lateral geniculate body).

IV   THE INTERNAL CAPSULE (Figure 17-2) is a layer of white matter (myelinated axons) that separates the caudate nucleus and the thalamus medially from the lentiform nucleus laterally.

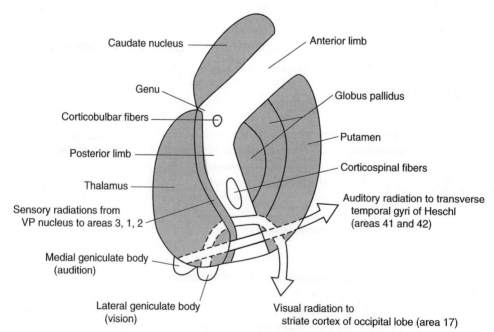

Figure 17-2 Horizontal section of the right internal capsule showing the major fiber projections. Clinically important tracts lie in the genu and posterior limb. Lesions of the internal capsule cause contralateral hemiparesis and contralateral hemianopia. *VP*, ventral posterior.

A. The **anterior limb** is located between the caudate nucleus and the lentiform nucleus (globus pallidus and putamen).

B. The **genu** contains the corticonuclear fibers.

C. The **posterior limb** is located between the thalamus and the lentiform nucleus. It contains corticospinal (pyramid) fibers as well as sensory (pain, temperature, and touch), visual, and auditory radiations.

D. BLOOD SUPPLY
 1. The **anterior limb** is irrigated by the medial striate branches of the anterior cerebral artery and the lateral striate (lenticulostriate) branches of the middle cerebral artery.
 2. The **genu** is perfused either by direct branches from the internal carotid artery or by pallidal branches of the anterior choroidal artery.
 3. The **posterior limb** is supplied by branches of the anterior choroidal artery and lenticulostriate branches of the middle cerebral arteries.

Case Study

A 90-year-old woman complains of an intense burning sensation on the left side of her neck and upper limb. The patient has a history of high blood pressure and diabetes. What is the most likely diagnosis?

Differentials
- Hypoglycemia; middle cerebral artery stroke; migraine

Relevant Physical Exam Findings
- Unilateral sensory loss is observed. Though the patient may complain of weakness on the affected side, no weakness is found on examination.

Relevant Lab Findings
- Normal serum glucose levels
- Thrombocytopenia
- Ischemic infarction of posterior cerebral artery seen on computed tomography scan

Diagnosis
- Infarction of the ventral posterolateral nucleus of the thalamus results in pure hemisensory loss contralateral to the lesion. → *Dejerine Roussy Syndrome.*

Chapter 18

Hypothalamus

 Key Concepts

1) Figures 18-1 and 18-2 show that the paraventricular and supraoptic nuclei synthesize and release antidiuretic hormone and oxytocin.
2) The suprachiasmatic nucleus receives direct input from the retina and plays a role in the regulation of circadian rhythms.

I INTRODUCTION

A. **GENERAL STRUCTURE AND FUNCTION.** The hypothalamus is a **division of the diencephalon** that subserves three systems: the autonomic nervous system, the endocrine system, and the limbic system. The hypothalamus helps to maintain homeostasis.

B. **MAJOR HYPOTHALAMIC NUCLEI AND THEIR FUNCTIONS**
 1. The **medial preoptic nucleus** (Figure 18-1) regulates the release of gonadotropic hormones from the adenohypophysis. It contains the sexually dimorphic nucleus, the development of which depends on testosterone levels.
 2. The **suprachiasmatic nucleus** receives direct input from the retina. It plays a role in the regulation of circadian rhythms.
 3. The **anterior nucleus** plays a role in temperature regulation. It stimulates the parasympathetic nervous system. Destruction results in hyperthermia.
 4. The **paraventricular nucleus** (Figure 18-2) synthesizes antidiuretic hormone (ADH), oxytocin, and corticotropin-releasing hormone. It gives rise to the supraopticohypophyseal tract, which projects to the neurohypophysis. It regulates water balance (conservation) and projects directly to the autonomic nuclei of the brain stem and all levels of the spinal cord. Destruction results in diabetes insipidus.
 5. The **supraoptic nucleus** synthesizes ADH and oxytocin (similar to the paraventricular nucleus).
 6. The **dorsomedial nucleus**, when stimulated in animals, results in savage behavior.
 7. The **ventromedial nucleus** is considered a satiety center. When stimulated, it inhibits the urge to eat. Bilateral destruction results in hyperphagia, obesity, and savage behavior.
 8. The **arcuate (infundibular) nucleus** contains neurons that produce factors that stimulate or inhibit the action of the hypothalamus. This nucleus gives rise to the tuberohypophysial tract, which terminates in the hypophyseal portal system (see Figure 18-2) of the infundibulum (medium eminence). It contains neurons that produce dopamine (i.e., prolactin-inhibiting factor).

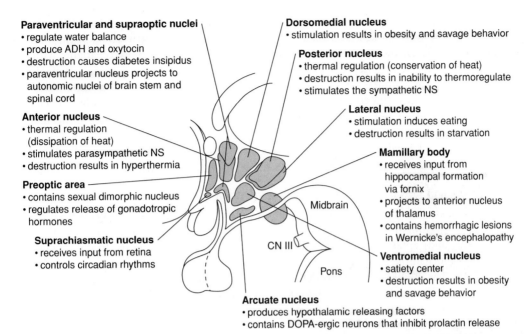

Paraventricular and supraoptic nuclei
- regulate water balance
- produce ADH and oxytocin
- destruction causes diabetes insipidus
- paraventricular nucleus projects to autonomic nuclei of brain stem and spinal cord

Anterior nucleus
- thermal regulation (dissipation of heat)
- stimulates parasympathetic NS
- destruction results in hyperthermia

Preoptic area
- contains sexual dimorphic nucleus
- regulates release of gonadotropic hormones

Suprachiasmatic nucleus
- receives input from retina
- controls circadian rhythms

Dorsomedial nucleus
- stimulation results in obesity and savage behavior

Posterior nucleus
- thermal regulation (conservation of heat)
- destruction results in inability to thermoregulate
- stimulates the sympathetic NS

Lateral nucleus
- stimulation induces eating
- destruction results in starvation

Mamillary body
- receives input from hippocampal formation via fornix
- projects to anterior nucleus of thalamus
- contains hemorrhagic lesions in Wernicke's encephalopathy

Ventromedial nucleus
- satiety center
- destruction results in obesity and savage behavior

Midbrain

CN III

Pons

Arcuate nucleus
- produces hypothalamic releasing factors
- contains DOPA-ergic neurons that inhibit prolactin release

Figure 18-1 Major hypothalamic nuclei and their functions. *ADH*, antidiuretic hormone; *CN*, cranial nerve; *DOPA*, dopamine; *NS*, nervous system.

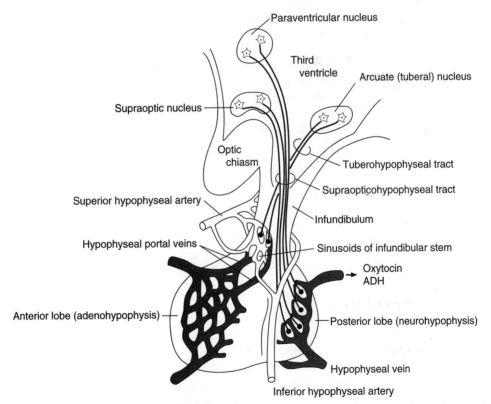

Paraventricular nucleus

Third ventricle

Arcuate (tuberal) nucleus

Supraoptic nucleus

Optic chiasm

Superior hypophyseal artery

Hypophyseal portal veins

Anterior lobe (adenohypophysis)

Tuberohypophyseal tract

Supraopticohypophyseal tract

Infundibulum

Sinusoids of infundibular stem

Oxytocin
ADH

Posterior lobe (neurohypophysis)

Hypophyseal vein

Inferior hypophyseal artery

Figure 18-2 The hypophyseal portal system. The paraventricular and supraoptic nuclei produce antidiuretic hormone (*ADH*) and oxytocin and transport them through the supraopticohypophysial tract to the capillary bed of the neurohypophysis. The arcuate nucleus of the infundibulum transports hypothalamic-stimulating hormones through the tuberohypophysial tract to the sinusoids of the infundibular stem. These sinusoids then drain into the secondary capillary plexus in the adenohypophysis.

9. The **mamillary nucleus** receives input from the hippocampal formation through the postcommissural fornix. It projects to the anterior nucleus of the thalamus through the mamillothalamic tract (part of the Papez circuit). Patients with Wernicke's encephalopathy, which is a thiamine (vitamin B_1) deficiency, have lesions in the mamillary nucleus. Lesions are also associated with alcoholism.

10. The **posterior hypothalamic nucleus** plays a role in thermal regulation (i.e., conservation and increased production of heat). Lesions result in **poikilothermia** (i.e., inability to thermoregulate).

11. The **lateral hypothalamic nucleus** induces eating when stimulated. **Lesions** cause **anorexia** and **starvation**.

C. MAJOR FIBER SYSTEMS OF THE HYPOTHALAMUS

1. The **fornix** is the largest projection to the hypothalamus. It projects from the hippocampal formation to the mamillary nucleus, anterior nucleus of the thalamus, and septal area. The fornix then projects from the septal area to the hippocampal formation.

2. The **medial forebrain bundle** traverses the entire lateral hypothalamic area. It interconnects the orbitofrontal cortex, septal area, hypothalamus, and midbrain.

3. The **mamillothalamic tract** projects from the mamillary nuclei to the anterior nucleus of the thalamus (part of the Papez circuit).

4. The **stria terminalis** is the major pathway from the amygdala. It interconnects the septal area, hypothalamus, and amygdala.

5. The **supraopticohypophysial tract** conducts fibers from the supraoptic and paraventricular nuclei to the neurohypophysis, which is the release site for ADH and oxytocin.

6. The **tuberohypophysial (tuberoinfundibular) tract** conducts fibers from the arcuate nucleus to the hypophyseal portal system (see Figure 18-2).

7. The **hypothalamospinal tract** contains direct descending autonomic fibers. These fibers influence the preganglionic sympathetic neurons of the intermediolateral cell column and preganglionic neurons of the sacral parasympathetic nucleus. Interruption above the first thoracic segment (T-1) causes Horner's syndrome.

II FUNCTIONS

A. AUTONOMIC FUNCTION

1. The **anterior hypothalamus** has an excitatory effect on the parasympathetic nervous system.

2. The **posterior hypothalamus** has an excitatory effect on the sympathetic nervous system.

B. TEMPERATURE REGULATION

1. The **anterior hypothalamus** regulates and maintains body temperature. Destruction causes hyperthermia.

2. The **posterior hypothalamus** helps to produce and conserve heat. Destruction causes the inability to thermoregulate.

C. WATER BALANCE REGULATION. The **paraventricular nucleus** synthesizes ADH, which controls water excretion by the kidneys.

D. FOOD INTAKE REGULATION. Two hypothalamic nuclei play a role in the control of appetite.

   1. When stimulated, the **ventromedial nucleus** inhibits the urge to eat. Bilateral destruction results in hyperphagia, obesity, and savage behavior.
   2. When stimulated, the **lateral hypothalamic nucleus** induces the urge to eat. Destruction causes starvation and emaciation.

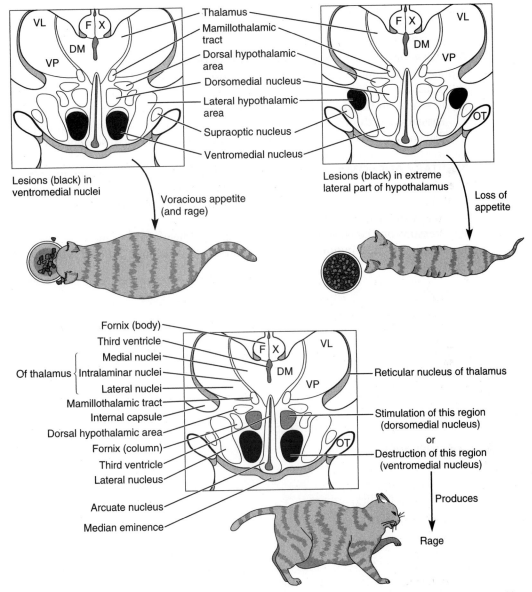

Figure 18-3 Coronal section through the hypothalamus at the level of the dorsomedial, ventromedial, and lateral hypothalamic nuclei. Lesions or stimulation of these nuclei result in obesity, cachexia, and rage. The column of the fornix separates the medial from the lateral hypothalamic zones. A lesion of the optic tract results in a contralateral hemianopia. *FX*, fornix; *DM*, medial dorsal nucleus of thalamus; *OT*, optic tract; *VL*, ventral lateral nucleus of thalamus; *VP*, ventral posterior nucleus of thalamus. (Reprinted from JD Fix, *BRS neuroanatomy*, 3rd ed. Baltimore: Williams & Wilkins, 1996:313, with permission.)

Ⅲ CLINICAL CORRELATION

A. DIABETES INSIPIDUS, which is characterized by polyuria and polydipsia, is the best-known hypothalamic syndrome. It results from lesions of the ADH pathways to the posterior lobe of the pituitary gland.

B. The **syndrome of inappropriate ADH secretion** is usually caused by lung tumors or drug therapy (e.g., carbamazepine, chlorpromazine).

C. CRANIOPHARYNGIOMA is a congenital tumor that originates from remnants of Rathke's pouch (see Chapter 1). This tumor is usually calcified. It is the most common supratentorial tumor in children and the most common cause of hypopituitarism in children.
   1. **Pressure on the chiasma** results in bitemporal hemianopia.
   2. **Pressure on the hypothalamus** causes hypothalamic syndrome (i.e., adiposity, diabetes insipidus, disturbance of temperature regulation, and somnolence).

D. PITUITARY ADENOMAS account for 15% of clinical symptomatic intracranial tumors. They are rarely seen in children. When pituitary adenomas are endocrine-active, they cause endocrine abnormalities (e.g., amenorrhea and galactorrhea from a prolactin-secreting adenoma, the most common type).
   1. **Pressure on the chiasma** results in bitemporal hemianopia.
   2. **Pressure on the hypothalamus** may cause hypothalamus syndrome (Figure 18-3).

Case Study

A 65-year-old diabetic man was hospitalized after an auto accident with lethargy and progressive confusion. Laboratory tests results revealed low sodium levels. The patient was discharged after serum sodium levels were elevated to 130 mmol/L.

Differentials

• Diabetes

Relevant Physical Exam Findings

• Fatigue and depression
• Slowed mental processing time
• Slowed pulse and hypothermia
• Hyporeflexia and hypotonia

Relevant Lab Findings

• Normal hepatic, renal, and cardiac function
• Hyponatremia that worsens with fluid load
• Serum hypoosmolality
• Urine hyperosmolarity

Diagnosis

• Inappropriate secretion of antidiuretic hormone by the hypothalamus. As many as 50% of traumatic brain injury patients experience endocrine complications that may result in intracerebral osmotic fluid shifts and brain edema, affecting hypothalamic function.

Chapter 19

Limbic System

 Key Concepts

1) Bilateral lesions of the amygdala result in Klüver-Bucy syndrome. Recall the triad hyperphagia, hypersexuality, and psychic blindness.
2) Memory loss is associated with bilateral lesions of the hippocampus.
3) Wernicke's encephalopathy results from a deficiency of thiamine (vitamin B_1). Lesions are found in the mamillary bodies, thalamus, and midbrain tegmentum (Figure 19-3).
4) Know the Papez circuit, a common board question.

I   INTRODUCTION   The limbic system is considered the anatomic substrate that underlies behavioral and emotional expression. It is expressed through the hypothalamus by way of the autonomic nervous system.

II   MAJOR COMPONENTS AND CONNECTIONS

A. The **orbitofrontal cortex** mediates the conscious perception of smell. It has reciprocal connections with the mediodorsal nucleus of the thalamus. It is interconnected through the medial forebrain bundle with the septal area and hypothalamic nuclei.

B. The **dorsomedial mediodorsal nucleus of the thalamus** has reciprocal connections with the orbitofrontal and prefrontal cortices and the hypothalamus. It receives input from the amygdala and plays a role in affective behavior and memory.

C. The **anterior nucleus of the thalamus** receives input from the mamillary nucleus through the mamillothalamic tract and fornix. It projects to the cingulate gyrus and is a major link in the Papez circuit.

D. The **septal area** is a telencephalic structure. It has reciprocal connections with the hippocampal formation through the fornix and with the hypothalamus through the medial forebrain bundle. It projects through the stria medullaris (thalami) to the habenular nucleus.

E. The **limbic lobe** includes the subcallosal area, paraterminal gyrus, cingulate gyrus and isthmus, and parahippocampal gyrus, which includes the uncus. It contains, buried in the parahippocampal gyrus, the hippocampal formation and amygdaloid nuclear complex.

F. The **hippocampal formation** is a sheet of archicortex that is jelly-rolled into the parahippocampal gyrus. It functions in learning, memory, and recognition of novelty. It receives major input through the entorhinal cortex and projects major output through the fornix. Its **major structures include the following:**

1. The **dentate gyrus**, which has a three-layered archicortex. It contains granule cells that receive hippocampal input and project output to the pyramidal cells of the hippocampus and subiculum.

2. The **hippocampus (cornu Ammonis)**, which has a three-layered archicortex. It contains pyramidal cells that project through the fornix to the septal area and hypothalamus.

3. The **subiculum**, which receives input through the hippocampal pyramidal cells. It projects through the fornix to the mamillary nuclei and the anterior nucleus of the thalamus.

G. The **amygdaloid complex (amygdala)** (Figure 19-1; see also Figure 21-1) is a basal nucleus that underlies the parahippocampal uncus. In humans, stimulation causes fear and signs of sympathetic overactivity. In other animals, stimulation results in cessation of activity and heightened attentiveness. Lesions cause placidity and hypersexual behavior.

1. **Input** is from the sensory association cortices, olfactory bulb and cortex, hypothalamus and septal area, and hippocampal formation.

2. **Output** is through the stria terminalis to the hypothalamus and septal area. There is also output to the dorsomedial nucleus of the thalamus.

H. The **hypothalamus** has reciprocal connections with the amygdala.

I. The **limbic midbrain nuclei** and **associated neurotransmitters** include the ventral tegmental area (**dopamine**), raphe nuclei (**serotonin**), and locus ceruleus (**norepinephrine**).

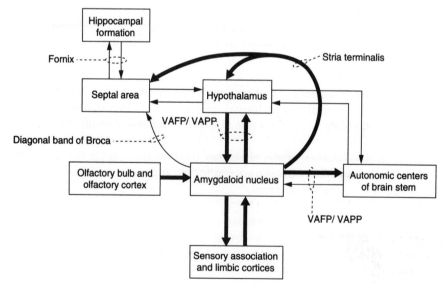

Figure 19-1 Major connections of the amygdaloid nucleus. This nucleus receives input from three major sources: the olfactory system, sensory association and limbic cortices, and hypothalamus. Major output is through two channels: The stria terminalis projects to the hypothalamus and the septal area, and the ventral amygdalofugal pathway (*VAFP*) projects to the hypothalamus, brain stem, and spinal cord. A smaller efferent bundle, the diagonal band of Broca, projects to the septal area. Afferent fibers from the hypothalamus and brain stem enter the amygdaloid nucleus through the ventral amygdalopetal pathway (*VAPP*).

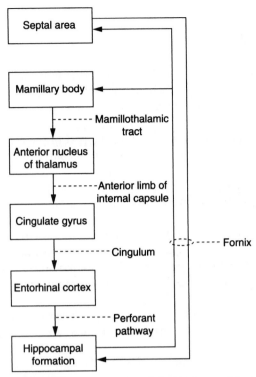

Figure 19-2 Major afferent and efferent limbic connections of the hippocampal formation. This formation has three components: the hippocampus (cornu Ammonis), subiculum, and dentate gyrus. The hippocampus projects to the septal area, the subiculum projects to the mamillary nuclei, and the dentate gyrus does not project beyond the hippocampal formation. The circuit of Papez follows this route: hippocampal formation to mamillary nucleus to anterior thalamic nucleus to cingulate gyrus to entorhinal cortex to hippocampal formation.

III **THE PAPEZ CIRCUIT** (Figure 19-2) includes the following limbic structures:

A. The **hippocampal formation**, which projects through the fornix to the mamillary nucleus and septal area.

B. The **mamillary nucleus.**

C. The **anterior thalamic nucleus.**

D. The **cingulate gyrus** (Brodmann's areas 23 and 24).

E. The **entorhinal area** (Brodmann's area 28).

IV **CLINICAL CORRELATION**

A. **KLÜVER-BUCY SYNDROME** results from bilateral ablation of the anterior temporal lobes, including the amygdaloid nuclei. It causes psychic blindness (visual agnosia), hyperphagia, docility (placidity), and hypersexuality.

B. **AMNESTIC (CONFABULATORY) SYNDROME** results from bilateral infarction of the hippocampal formation (i.e., hippocampal branches of the posterior cerebral arteries and anterior choroidal arteries of the internal carotid arteries). It causes anterograde amnesia (i.e., inability to learn and retain new information). **Memory loss suggests hippocampal pathology.**

C. FOSTER KENNEDY SYNDROME results from **meningioma** of the **olfactory groove.** The meningioma compresses the olfactory tract and optic nerve. Ipsilateral anosmia and optic atrophy and contralateral papilledema occur as a result of increased intracranial pressure.

D. The **hippocampus** is the most epileptogenic part of the cerebrum. Lesions may cause psychomotor attacks. Sommer's sector is very sensitive to ischemia.

E. Bilateral transection of the fornix may cause the acute amnestic syndrome (i.e., inability to consolidate short-term memory into long-term memory).

F. WERNICKE'S ENCEPHALOPATHY results from a thiamine (vitamin B_1) deficiency. The clinical triad includes ocular disturbances and nystagmus, gait ataxia, and mental dysfunction. Pathologic features include mamillary nuclei, dorsomedial nuclei of the thalamus, and periaqueductal gray and pontine tegmentum (Figure 19-3).

G. STRACHAN'S SYNDROME results from high-dose thiamine (vitamin B_1) therapy. The clinical triad includes spinal ataxia, optic atrophy, and nerve deafness.

H. Bilateral destruction or removal of the cingulate gyri causes loss of initiative and inhibition and dulling of the emotions. Memory is unaffected. Lesions of the anterior cingulate gyri cause placidity. Cingulectomy is used to treat severe anxiety and depression (Figure 19-4).

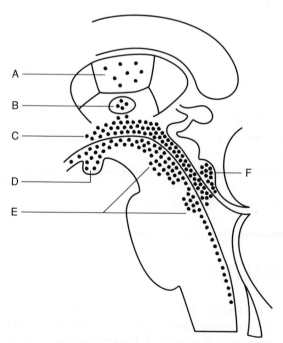

Figure 19-3 Midsagittal section through the brain stem and diencephalon showing the distribution of lesions in Wernicke's encephalopathy. (*A*) Dorsomedial nucleus of the thalamus. (*B*) Massa intermedia. (*C*) Periventricular area. (*D*) Mamillary nuclei. (*E*) Midbrain and pontine tegmentum. (*F*) Inferior colliculus. Lesions in the mamillary nuclei are associated with Wernicke's encephalopathy and thiamine (vitamin B_1) deficiency.

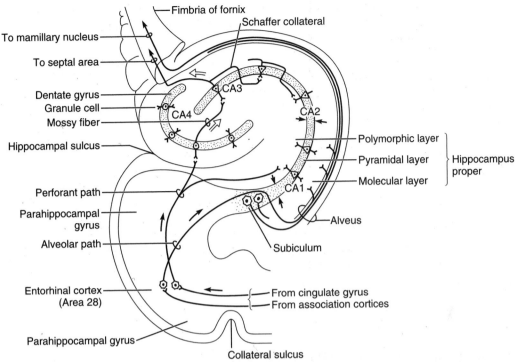

Figure 19-4 Major connections of the hippocampal formation. The hippocampal formation (HF) consists of three parts: hippocampus, dentate gyrus, and subiculum. The two major hypothalamic output pathways are (1) granule cell via mossy fiber to pyramidal cell via precommissural fornix to septal nuclei and (2) subicular neuron via postcommissural fornix to the medial mamillary nucleus. The HF plays an important role in learning and memory, and lesions of the HF result in short-term memory defects. In Alzheimer's disease, loss of cells in the HF and entorhinal cortex leads to loss of memory and cognitive function. *CA*, cornu ammonis. The sector CA1 is very sensitive to hypoxia (cardiac arrest or stroke). (Reprinted from JD Fix, *BRS neuroanatomy*, 3rd ed. Baltimore: Williams & Wilkins, 1996:332, with permission.)

Case Study

A 15-year-old boy was knocked out after several rounds of boxing with friends. Computed tomography scanning showed acute subdural hematoma associated with the right cerebral hemisphere. After regaining consciousness, the boy no longer experienced normal fear and anger and demonstrated aberrant sexual behaviors and excessive oral tendencies. He also complained of being very hungry all the time. What is the most likely diagnosis?

Relevant Lab Findings

- Computed tomography and magnetic resonance imaging revealed lesions of the right temporal lobe and right-dominant orbitofrontal regions, including bilateral rectal and medial orbital gyri, and an intact left temporal lobe.

Diagnosis

- Klüver-Bucy syndrome occurs when both the right and left medial temporal lobes malfunction, with frequent involvement of the amygdala. The cardinal symptom is excessive oral tendencies where the patient puts all types of objects into the mouth. Such patients also have an irresistible impulse to touch objects and demonstrate placidity (lack of emotional response) and a marked increase in sexual activity, without concern for social appropriateness.

Chapter 20

Cerebellum

 Key Concepts

1) Figure 20-1 shows the most important cerebellar circuit.
2) The inhibitory γ-aminobutyric acid (GABA)-ergic cerebellar output is regulated by Purkinje.
3) Purkinje cells give rise to the cerebellodentatothalamic tract.
4) What are mossy and climbing fibers?

I FUNCTION
The cerebellum has three primary functions:

A. MAINTENANCE OF POSTURE AND BALANCE

B. MAINTENANCE OF MUSCLE TONE

C. COORDINATION OF VOLUNTARY MOTOR ACTIVITY

II ANATOMY

A. CEREBELLAR PEDUNCLES
1. The **superior cerebellar peduncle** contains the major output from the cerebellum, the dentatothalamic tract. This tract terminates in the ventral lateral nucleus of the thalamus. It has one major afferent pathway, the ventral spinocerebellar tract.
2. The **middle cerebellar peduncle** receives pontocerebellar fibers, which project to the neocerebellum (pontocerebellum).
3. The **inferior cerebellar peduncle** has three major afferent tracts: the dorsal spinocerebellar tract, the cuneocerebellar tract, and the olivocerebellar tract from the contralateral inferior olivary nucleus.

B. CEREBELLAR CORTEX, NEURONS, AND FIBERS
1. **The cerebellar cortex has three layers.**
   a. The **molecular layer** is the outer layer underlying the pia. It contains stellate cells, basket cells, and the dendritic arbor of the Purkinje cells.
   b. The **Purkinje cell layer** lies between the molecular and the granule cell layers.
   c. The **granule layer** is the inner layer overlying the white matter. It contains granule cells, Golgi cells, and cerebellar glomeruli. A cerebellar glomerulus consists of a mossy fiber rosette, granule cell dendrites, and a Golgi cell axon.
2. **Neurons and fibers of the cerebellum**
   a. **Purkinje cells** convey the only output from the cerebellar cortex. They project inhibitory output [i.e., γ-aminobutyric acid (GABA)] to the cerebellar and

vestibular nuclei. These cells are excited by parallel and climbing fibers and inhibited by GABAergic basket and stellate cells.

b. **Granule cells** excite (by way of glutamate) Purkinje, basket, stellate, and Golgi cells through parallel fibers. They are inhibited by Golgi cells and excited by mossy fibers.

c. **Parallel fibers** are the axons of granule cells. These fibers extend into the molecular layer.

d. **Mossy fibers** are the afferent excitatory fibers of the spinocerebellar, ponto-cerebellar, and vestibulocerebellar tracts. They terminate as mossy fiber rosettes on granule cell dendrites. They excite granule cells to discharge through their parallel fibers.

e. **Climbing fibers** are the afferent excitatory (by way of aspartate) fibers of the olivo-cerebellar tract. These fibers arise from the contralateral inferior olivary nucleus. They terminate on neurons of the cerebellar nuclei and dendrites of Purkinje cells.

III THE MAJOR CEREBELLAR PATHWAY (Figure 20-1) consists of the following structures.

A. The **Purkinje cells of the cerebellar cortex** project to the cerebellar nuclei (e.g., dentate, emboliform, globose, and fastigial nuclei).

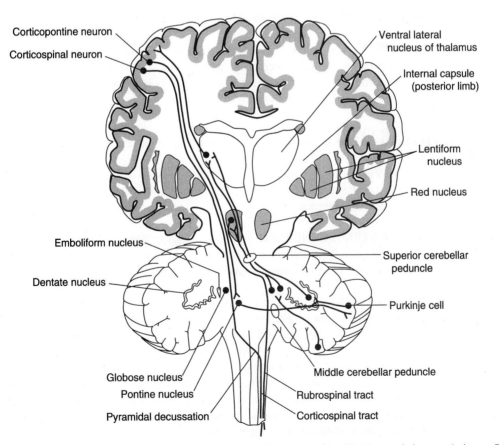

Figure 20-1 The principal cerebellar connections. The major efferent pathway is the dentatothalamocortical tract. The cerebellum receives input from the cerebral cortex through the corticopontocerebellar tract.

B. The **dentate nucleus** is the major effector nucleus of the cerebellum. It gives rise to the **dentatothalamic tract**, which projects through the superior cerebellar peduncle to the contralateral ventral lateral nucleus of the thalamus. The decussation of the superior cerebellar peduncle is in the caudal midbrain tegmentum.

C. The **ventral lateral nucleus of the thalamus** receives the dentatothalamic tract. It projects to the primary motor cortex of the precentral gyrus (Brodmann's area 4).

D. The **motor cortex (motor strip, or Brodmann's area 4)** receives input from the ventral lateral nucleus of the thalamus. It projects as the corticopontine tract to the pontine nuclei.

E. The **pontine nuclei** receive input from the motor cortex. Axons project as the pontocerebellar tract to the contralateral cerebellar cortex, where they terminate as mossy fibers, thus completing the circuit.

IV CEREBELLAR DYSFUNCTION includes the following triad:

A. HYPOTONIA is loss of the resistance normally offered by muscles to palpation or passive manipulation. It results in a floppy, loose-jointed, rag-doll appearance with pendular reflexes. The patient appears inebriated.

B. DYSEQUILIBRIUM is loss of balance characterized by gait and trunk dystaxia.

C. DYSSYNERGIA is loss of coordinated muscle activity. It includes **dysmetria, intention tremor, failure to check movements, nystagmus, dysdiadochokinesia,** and **dysrhythmokinesia. Cerebellar nystagmus is coarse. It is more pronounced when the patient looks toward the side of the lesion.**

V CEREBELLAR SYNDROMES AND TUMORS (Figure 20-2)

A. ANTERIOR VERMIS SYNDROME involves the leg region of the anterior lobe. It results from atrophy of the rostral vermis, most commonly caused by alcohol abuse. It causes gait, trunk, and leg dystaxia.

B. POSTERIOR VERMIS SYNDROME involves the flocculonodular lobe. It is usually the result of brain tumors in children and is most commonly caused by medulloblastomas or ependymomas. It causes truncal dystaxia.

C. HEMISPHERIC SYNDROME usually involves one cerebellar hemisphere. It is often the result of a brain tumor (astrocytoma) or an abscess (secondary to otitis media or mastoiditis). It causes arm, leg, and gait dystaxia and ipsilateral cerebellar signs.

D. CEREBELLAR TUMORS. In children, 70% of brain tumors are found in the posterior fossa. In adults, 70% of brain tumors are found in the supratentorial compartment.
   1. **Astrocytomas** constitute 30% of all brain tumors in children. They are most often found in the cerebellar hemisphere. After surgical removal of an astrocytoma, it is common for the child to survive for many years.
   2. **Medulloblastomas** are malignant and constitute 20% of all brain tumors in children. They are believed to originate from the superficial granule layer of the cerebellar cortex. They usually obstruct the passage of cerebrospinal fluid (CSF). As a result, hydrocephalus occurs.

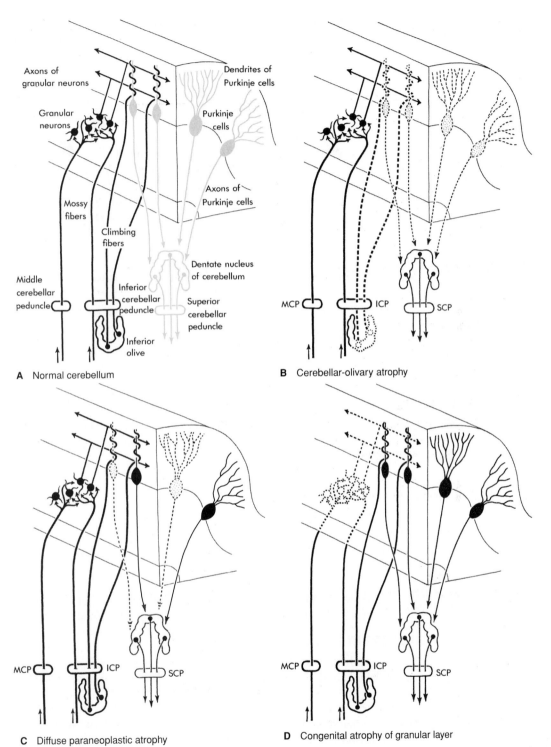

A Normal cerebellum

B Cerebellar-olivary atrophy

C Diffuse paraneoplastic atrophy

D Congenital atrophy of granular layer

Figure 20-2 Various forms of cerebellar atrophy. *MCP*, middle cerebellar peduncle; *ICP*, inferior cerebellar peduncle; *SCP*, superior cerebellar peduncle. (Reprinted from J Poirier, F Gray, R Escourolle, *Manual of basic neuropathology*, 3rd ed. Philadelphia: WB Saunders, 1990:155, with permission.) *(continued)*

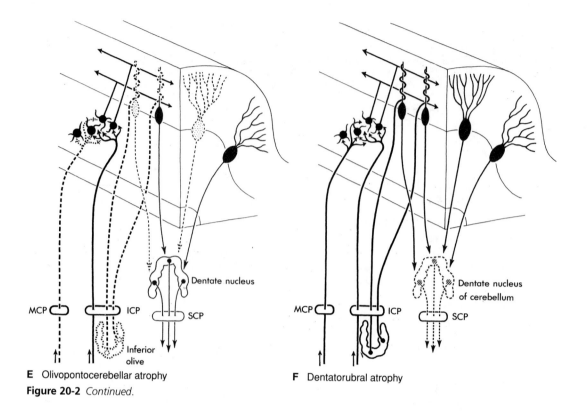

E Olivopontocerebellar atrophy

F Dentatorubral atrophy

Figure 20-2 *Continued.*

3. **Ependymomas** constitute 15% of all brain tumors in children. They occur most frequently in the fourth ventricle. They usually obstruct the passage of CSF and cause hydrocephalus.

Case Study

A 50-year-old woman presented with a history of poor coordination of hands, speech, and eye movements, accompanied by personality changes and some deterioration of intellectual function.

Relevant Physical Exam Findings

• Neurologic examination revealed marked cerebellar ataxia and spasticity of all extremities, held in a flexed posture. Babinski's sign was negative. The sensory system appeared normal.

Relevant Lab Findings

• Laboratory results were unremarkable. A brain computed tomography scan showed generalized cerebral atrophy, most pronounced in the cerebellum.

Diagnosis

• Spinocerebellar ataxia is a genetic disease that is characterized by progressive loss of coordination of gait, with frequent involvement of hands, speech, and eye movements. At least 29 different gene mutations have been associated with the various forms of this disease.

Chapter **21**

Basal Nuclei (Ganglia) and Striatal Motor System

Key Concepts

1) Figure 21-6 shows the circuitry of the basal ganglia and their associated neurotransmitters.
2) Parkinson's disease is associated with a depopulation of neurons in the substantia nigra.
3) Huntington's disease results in a loss of nerve cells in the caudate nucleus and putamen.
4) Hemiballism results from infarction of the contralateral subthalamic nucleus.

I BASAL NUCLEI (GANGLIA) (Figure 21-1)

A. COMPONENTS
1. **Caudate nucleus**
2. **Putamen**
3. **Globus pallidus**

B. GROUPING OF THE BASAL NUCLEI (GANGLIA)
1. The **striatum** consists of the caudate nucleus and putamen.
2. The **lentiform nucleus** consists of the globus pallidus and putamen.
3. The **corpus striatum** consists of the lentiform nucleus and caudate nucleus.
4. The **claustrum** lies between the lentiform nucleus and the insular cortex. It has reciprocal connections between the sensory cortices (i.e., visual cortex) (Figures 21-2 through 21-4).

II THE STRIATAL (EXTRAPYRAMIDAL) MOTOR SYSTEM (see Figure 21-1) plays
a role in the initiation and execution of somatic motor activity, especially willed movement. It is also involved in automatic stereotyped postural and reflex motor activity (e.g., normal subjects swing their arms when they walk).

A. STRUCTURE. The striatal motor system includes the following structures:
1. **Neocortex.**
2. **Striatum (caudatoputamen,** or **neostriatum).**
3. **Globus pallidus.**
4. **Subthalamic nucleus.**
5. **Substantia nigra** (i.e., pars compacta and pars reticularis).
6. **Thalamus** (ventral anterior, ventral lateral, and centromedian nuclei).

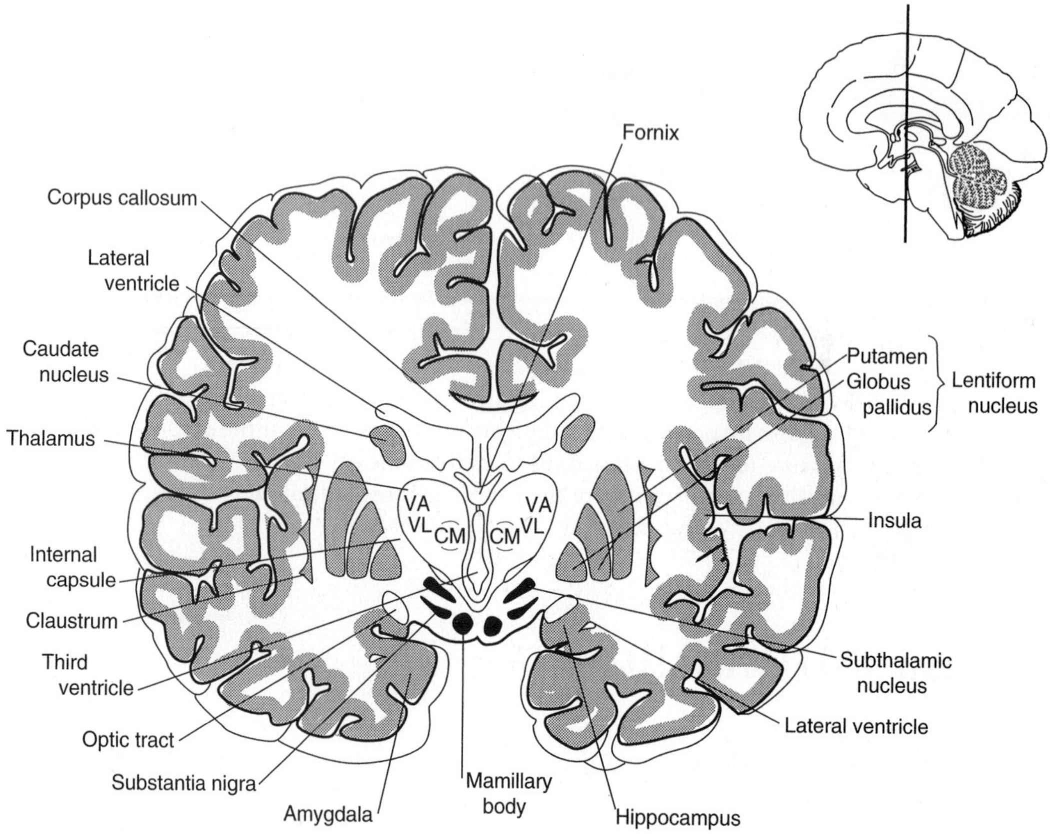

● **Figure 21-1** Coronal section through the midthalamus at the level of the mamillary bodies. The basal nuclei (ganglia) are all prominent at this level and include the striatum and lentiform nucleus. The subthalamic nucleus and substantia nigra are important components of the striatal motor system. *CM*, centromedian nucleus; *VA*, ventral anterior nucleus; *VL*, ventral lateral nucleus. (Modified from TA Woolsey, J Hanaway, MH Gado, *The brain atlas: a visual guide to the human central nervous system*, 2nd ed. Hoboken: John Wiley & Sons, 2003:68, with permission.)

B. Figure 21-5 shows the **major afferent** and **efferent connections** of the striatal system.

C. NEUROTRANSMITTERS are seen in Figure 21-6.

III CLINICAL CORRELATION

A. PARKINSON'S DISEASE. This is a **degenerative disease** that affects the substantia nigra and its projections to the striatum.

1. **RESULTS** of Parkinson's disease are a **depletion of dopamine** in the substantia nigra and striatum as well as a **loss of melanin-containing dopaminergic neurons** in the substantia nigra.
2. **CLINICAL SIGNS** are bradykinesia, stooped posture, shuffling gait, cogwheel rigidity, pill-rolling tremor, and masked facies. **Lewy bodies** are found in the melanin-containing neurons of the substantia nigra. **Progressive supranuclear palsy** is associated with Parkinson's disease.
3. **TREATMENT** has been successful with L-dopa. Surgical intervention includes **pallidotomy** (rigidity) and **ventral thalomotomy** (tremor).

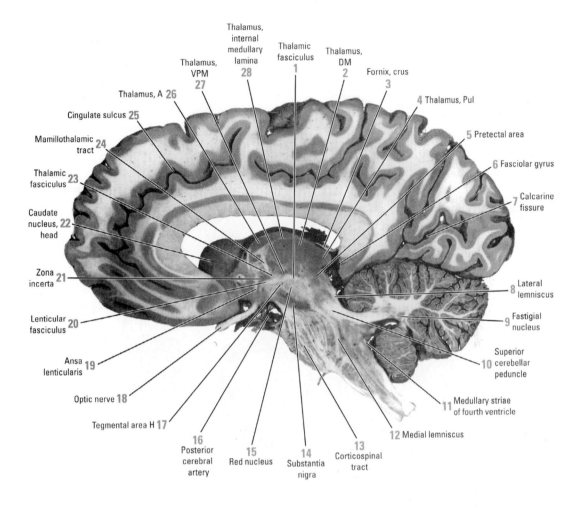

Thalamus, internal medullary lamina 28
Thalamus, VPM 27
Thalamus, A 26
Cingulate sulcus 25
Mamillothalamic tract 24
Thalamic fasciculus 23
Caudate nucleus, 22 head
Zona incerta 21
Lenticular fasciculus 20
Ansa lenticularis 19
Optic nerve 18
Tegmental area H 17
16 Posterior cerebral artery
15 Red nucleus
14 Substantia nigra
13 Corticospinal tract
Thalamic fasciculus 1
Thalamus, DM 2
Fornix, crus 3
4 Thalamus, Pul
5 Pretectal area
6 Fasciolar gyrus
7 Calcarine fissure
8 Lateral lemniscus
9 Fastigial nucleus
10 Superior cerebellar peduncle
11 Medullary striae of fourth ventricle
12 Medial lemniscus

Ansa lenticularis 19
Calcarine fissure 7
Caudate nucleus, head 22
Cingulate sulcus 25
Corticospinal (pyramidal) tract 13
Fasciolar gyrus 6
Fastigial nucleus 9
Fornix, crus 3
Lateral lemniscus 8
Lenticular fasciculus (H₂ field of *Forel*) 20

Mamillothalamic tract 24
Medial lemniscus 12
Medullary striae of fourth ventricle (IV) 11
Optic nerve (CN II) 18
Posterior cerebral artery 16
Pretectal area 5
Red nucleus 15
Substantia nigra 14
Superior cerebellar peduncle (brachium conjunctivum) 10

Tegmental area H (H field of *Forel*) 17
Thalamic fasciculus (H₁ field of *Forel*) 1, 23
Thalamus, anterior nucleus (A) 26
Thalamus, dorsomedial nucleus (DM) 2
Thalamus, internal medullary lamina 28
Thalamus, pulvinar (Pul) 4
Thalamus, ventroposteromedial nucleus (VPM) 27
Zona incerta 21

● **Figure 21-2** A parasagittal section through the caudate nucleus (*5*) and the substantia nigra (*10*): subthalamic nucleus (*11*), internal capsule (*12*), thalamus (*13*), cingulate gyrus (*14*). (Modified from TA Woolsey, J Hanaway, MH Gado, *The brain atlas: a visual guide to the human central nervous system*, 2nd ed. Hoboken: John Wiley & Sons, 2003:128, with permission.)

B. METHYLPHENYLTETRAHYDROPYRIDINE (MPTP)-INDUCED PARKINSONISM. MPTP is an analog of meperidine (Demerol). It destroys dopaminergic neurons in the substantia nigra.

C. HUNTINGTON'S DISEASE (chorea). This is an **inherited autosomal dominant movement disorder** that is traced to a single gene defect on chromosome 4.
1. It is associated with **degeneration of the cholinergic and γ-aminobutyric acid (GABA)-ergic neurons** of the striatum. It is accompanied by gyral atrophy in the frontal and temporal lobes.

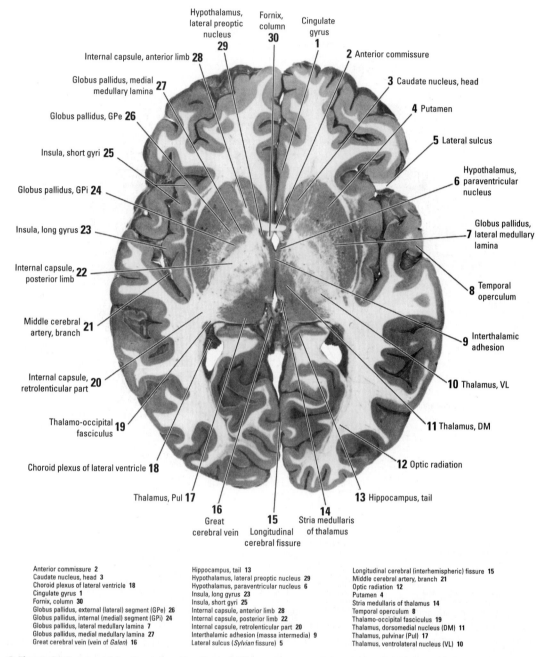

Hypothalamus, lateral preoptic nucleus **29**
Fornix, column **30**
Cingulate gyrus **1**

Internal capsule, anterior limb **28**

Globus pallidus, medial medullary lamina **27**

Globus pallidus, GPe **26**

Insula, short gyri **25**

Globus pallidus, GPi **24**

Insula, long gyrus **23**

Internal capsule, posterior limb **22**

Middle cerebral artery, branch **21**

Internal capsule, retrolenticular part **20**

Thalamo-occipital fasciculus **19**

Choroid plexus of lateral ventricle **18**

Thalamus, Pul **17**

16
Great cerebral vein

15
Longitudinal cerebral fissure

14
Stria medullaris of thalamus

13 Hippocampus, tail

2 Anterior commissure

3 Caudate nucleus, head

4 Putamen

5 Lateral sulcus

Hypothalamus, **6** paraventricular nucleus

Globus pallidus, **7** lateral medullary lamina

8 Temporal operculum

9 Interthalamic adhesion

10 Thalamus, VL

11 Thalamus, DM

12 Optic radiation

Anterior commissure **2**
Caudate nucleus, head **3**
Choroid plexus of lateral ventricle **18**
Cingulate gyrus **1**
Fornix, column **30**
Globus pallidus, external (lateral) segment (GPe) **26**
Globus pallidus, internal (medial) segment (GPi) **24**
Globus pallidus, lateral medullary lamina **7**
Globus pallidus, medial medullary lamina **27**
Great cerebral vein (vein of *Galen*) **16**

Hippocampus, tail **13**
Hypothalamus, lateral preoptic nucleus **29**
Hypothalamus, paraventricular nucleus **6**
Insula, long gyrus **23**
Insula, short gyri **25**
Internal capsule, anterior limb **28**
Internal capsule, posterior limb **22**
Internal capsule, retrolenticular part **20**
Interthalamic adhesion (massa intermedia) **9**
Lateral sulcus (*Sylvian* fissure) **5**

Longitudinal cerebral (interhispheric) fissure **15**
Middle cerebral artery, branch **21**
Optic radiation **12**
Putamen **4**
Stria medullaris of thalamus **14**
Temporal operculum **8**
Thalamo-occipital fasciculus **19**
Thalamus, dorsomedial nucleus (DM) **11**
Thalamus, pulvinar (Pul) **17**
Thalamus, ventrolateral nucleus (VL) **10**

● **Figure 21-3** An axial (horizontal) section through the anterior commissure (*15*) and the massa intermedia (*16*): internal capsule (*6*), globus pallidus (*7*), insular cortex (*14*), putamen (*17*), claustrum (*2*), head of caudate nucleus (*18*). (Modified from TA Woolsey, J Hanaway, MH Gado, *The brain atlas: a visual guide to the human central nervous system*, 2nd ed. Hoboken: John Wiley & Sons, 2003:100, with permission.)

2. **Glutamate (GLU) excitotoxicity** results when GLU is released in the striatum and binds to its receptors on striatal neurons, culminating in an action potential. GLU is removed from the extracellular space by astrocytes. In Huntington's disease, GLU is bound to the N-methyl-D-aspartate receptor, resulting in an influx of calcium ions and subsequent cell death. This cascade of events

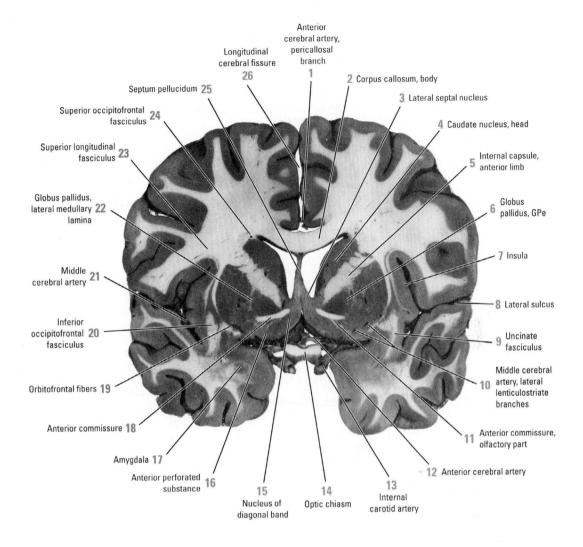

Anterior cerebral artery, pericallosal branch **1**

Longitudinal cerebral fissure **26**

Septum pellucidum **25**

Superior occipitofrontal fasciculus **24**

Superior longitudinal fasciculus **23**

Globus pallidus, lateral medullary lamina **22**

Middle cerebral artery **21**

Inferior occipitofrontal fasciculus **20**

Orbitofrontal fibers **19**

Anterior commissure **18**

Amygdala **17**

Anterior perforated substance **16**

15 Nucleus of diagonal band

14 Optic chiasm

13 Internal carotid artery

2 Corpus callosum, body

3 Lateral septal nucleus

4 Caudate nucleus, head

5 Internal capsule, anterior limb

6 Globus pallidus, GPe

7 Insula

8 Lateral sulcus

9 Uncinate fasciculus

10 Middle cerebral artery, lateral lenticulostriate branches

11 Anterior commissure, olfactory part

12 Anterior cerebral artery

Amygdala 17
Anterior cerebral artery 12
Anterior cerebral artery, pericallosal branch 1
Anterior commissure 18
Anterior commissure, olfactory part 11
Anterior perforated substance 16
Caudate nucleus, head 4
Corpus callosum, body 2
Globus pallidus, external (lateral) segment (GPe) 6
Globus pallidus, lateral medullary lamina 22

Inferior occipitofrontal fasciculus 20
Insula 7
Internal capsule, anterior limb 5
Internal carotid artery 13
Lateral septal nucleus 3
Lateral sulcus (*Sylvian* fissure) 8
Longitudinal cerebral (interhemispheric) fissure 26
Middle cerebral artery 21
Middle cerebral artery, lateral lenticulostriate branches [medial lenticulostriate branches originate from the anterior cerebral artery] 10

Nucleus of diagonal band (diagonal band of *Broca*) 15
Optic chiasm 14
Orbitofrontal fibers 19
Septum pellucidum 25
Superior longitudinal fasciculus 23
Superior occipitofrontal fasciculus 24
Uncinate fasciculus 9

● **Figure 21-4** A coronal section through the lentiform nucleus and the amygdaloid nucleus (*1*); the lentiform nucleus consists of the putamen (*8*) and the globus pallidus (*7*); the amygdaloid nucleus appears as a circular profile below the uncus. (Modified from TA Woolsey, J Hanaway, MH Gado, *The brain atlas: a visual guide to the human central nervous system*, 2nd ed. Hoboken: John Wiley & Sons, 2003:60, with permission.)

with neuronal death most likely occurs in cerebrovascular accidents (e.g., stroke).

3. **Clinical signs** include choreiform movements, hypotonia, and progressive dementia.

D. OTHER CHOREIFORM DYSKINESIAS

1. **Sydenham's chorea (St. Vitus' dance)** is the most common cause of chorea overall. It occurs primarily in girls, typically after a bout of rheumatic fever.

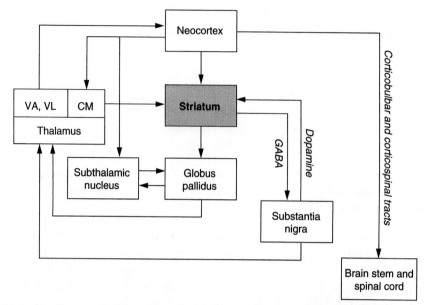

● **Figure 21-5** Major afferent and efferent connections of the striatal system. The striatum receives major input from three sources: the thalamus, neocortex, and substantia nigra. The striatum projects to the globus pallidus and substantia nigra. The globus pallidus is the effector nucleus of the striatal system; it projects to the thalamus and subthalamic nucleus. The substantia nigra also projects to the thalamus. The striatal motor system is expressed through the corticobulbar and corticospinal tracts. *CM*, centromedian nucleus; *GABA*, γ-aminobutyric acid; *VA*, ventral anterior nucleus; *VL*, ventral lateral nucleus.

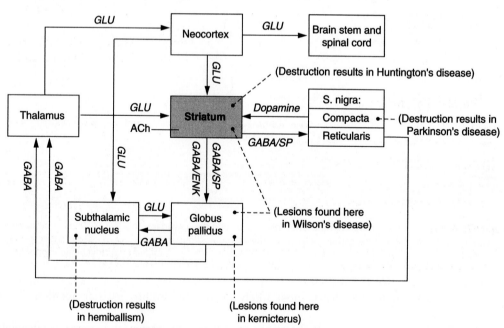

● **Figure 21-6** Major neurotransmitters of the striatal motor system. Within the striatum, globus pallidus, and pars reticularis of the substantia nigra (*S. nigra*), γ-aminobutyric acid (*GABA*) is the predominant neurotransmitter. GABA may coexist in the same neuron with enkephalin (*ENK*) or substance P (*SP*). Dopamine-containing neurons are found in the pars compacta of the substantia nigra. Acetylcholine (*ACh*) is found in the local circuit neurons of the striatum. The subthalamic nucleus projects excitatory glutaminergic fibers to the globus pallidus. *GLU*, glutamate.

2. **Chorea gravidarum** usually occurs during the second trimester of pregnancy. Many patients have a history of Sydenham's chorea.

E. **HEMIBALLISM** is a movement disorder that usually results from a vascular lesion of the subthalamic nucleus. Clinical signs include violent contralateral **flinging (ballistic) movements of one or both extremities.**

F. **HEPATOLENTICULAR DEGENERATION (WILSON'S DISEASE)** is an autosomal recessive disorder that is caused by a defect in the **metabolism of copper.** The gene locus is on chromosome 13.
   1. **Clinical signs** include choreiform or athetotic movements, rigidity, and **wing-beating tremor.** Tremor is the most common neurologic sign.
   2. **Lesions** are found in the **lentiform nucleus.** Copper deposition in the limbus of the cornea gives rise to the **corneal Kayser-Fleischer ring,** which is a pathognomonic sign. Deposition of copper in the liver leads to multilobar cirrhosis.
   3. **Psychiatric symptoms** include psychosis, personality disorders, and dementia.
   4. The **diagnosis** is based on low serum ceruloplasmin, elevated urinary excretion of copper, and increased copper concentration in a liver biopsy specimen.
   5. **Treatment** includes **penicillamine,** a **chelator.**

G. **TARDIVE DYSKINESIA** is a syndrome of **repetitive choreic movement** that **affects the face and trunk.** It results from treatment with phenothiazines, butyrophenones, or metoclopramide.

Case Study

A 30-year-old man presents with dysarthria, dysphagia, stiffness, and slow ataxic gait. There is no history of schizophrenia or depression and no family history of any neurodegenerative disease.

Relevant Physical Exam Findings
- The patient scored a 20/26 on the mini-mental status exam. The patient showed increased tone in all extremities, with normal strength.

Relevant Lab Findings
- A generalized cerebral and cerebellar atrophy and a very small caudate nucleus were revealed on magnetic resonance imaging scans.

Diagnosis
- Huntington's disease (chorea) is caused by a trinucleotide repeat in the gene coding for the Hungtinton protein. It is characterized by abnormal body movements and lack of coordination but can also affect mental abilities.

Chapter 22

Cerebral Cortex

✔ **Key Concepts**

1) This chapter describes the cortical localization of functional areas of the brain.
2) How does the dominant hemisphere differ from the nondominant hemisphere?
3) Figure 22-5 shows the effects of various major hemispheric lesions.
4) What symptoms result from a lesion of the right inferior parietal lobe?
5) What is Gerstmann's syndrome?

I   **INTRODUCTION**   The cerebral cortex, the thin, gray covering of both hemispheres of the brain, has two types: the neocortex (90%) and the allocortex (10%). Motor cortex is the thickest (4.5 mm); visual cortex is the thinnest (1.5 mm).

II   **THE SIX-LAYERED NEOCORTEX**   Layers II and IV of the neocortex are mainly afferent (i.e., receiving). Layers V and VI are mainly efferent (i.e., sending) (Figure 22-1).

A. LAYER I is the **molecular** layer.

B. LAYER II is the **external granular** layer.

C. LAYER III is the **external pyramidal** layer. It gives rise to association and commissural fibers and is the major source of corticocortical fibers.

D. LAYER IV is the **internal granular** layer. It receives thalamocortical fibers from the thalamic nuclei of the ventral tier (i.e., ventral posterolateral and ventral posteromedial). In the visual cortex (Brodmann's area 17), layer IV receives input from the lateral geniculate body.

E. LAYER V is the **internal pyramidal** layer. It gives rise to corticobulbar, corticospinal, and corticostriatal fibers. It contains the giant pyramidal cells of Betz, which are found only in the motor cortex (Brodmann's area 4).

F. LAYER VI is the **multiform** layer. It is the **major source of corticothalamic fibers**. It gives rise to projection, commissural, and association fibers.

III   **FUNCTIONAL AREAS** (Figure 22-2)

A. FRONTAL LOBE

    1. The **motor cortex** (Brodmann's area 4) and **premotor cortex** (Brodmann's area 6). These two cortices are somatotopically organized (Figure 22-3). Destruction

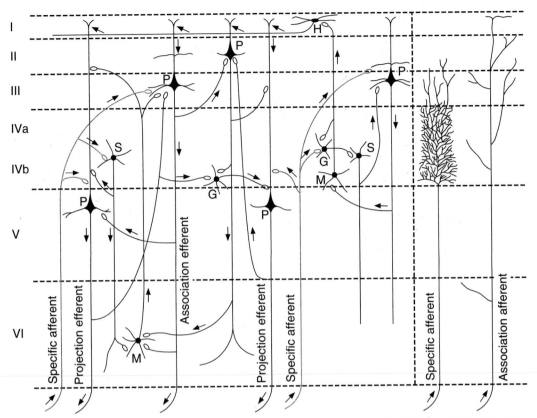

● **Figure 22-1** Neurocortical circuits. *G*, granule cell; *H*, horizontal cell; *M*, Martinotti cell; *P*, pyramidal cell; *S*, stellate cell. Loops show synaptic junctions. (Reprinted from A Parent, *Carpenter's human neuroanatomy*, 9th ed. Baltimore: Williams & Wilkins, 1996:868, with permission.)

of these areas of the frontal lobe causes contralateral spastic paresis. Contralateral pronator drift is associated with frontal lobe lesions of the corticospinal tract.

2. **Frontal eye field** (Brodmann's area 8). Destruction causes deviation of the eyes to the ipsilateral side.

3. **Broca's speech area** (Brodmann's areas 44 and 45). This is located in the posterior part of the inferior frontal gyrus in the dominant hemisphere (Figure 22-4). Destruction results in expressive, nonfluent aphasia (Broca's aphasia). The patient understands both written and spoken language but cannot articulate speech or write normally. Broca's aphasia is usually associated with contralateral facial and arm weakness because of the involvement of the motor strip.

4. **Prefrontal cortex** (Brodmann's areas 9–12 and 46–47). Destruction of the anterior two-thirds of the frontal lobe convexity results in deficits in concentration, orientation, abstracting ability, judgment, and problem-solving ability. Other frontal lobe deficits include loss of initiative, inappropriate behavior, release of sucking and grasping reflexes, gait apraxia, and sphincteric incontinence. Destruction of the orbital (frontal) lobe results in inappropriate social behavior (e.g., use of obscene language, urinating in public). Perseveration is associated with frontal lobe lesions.

A

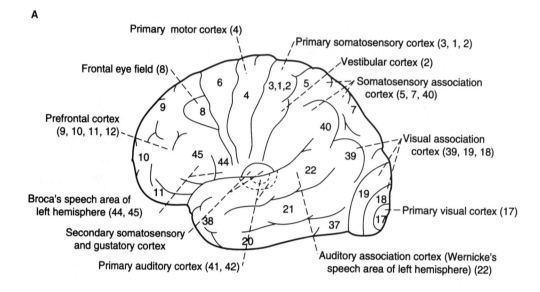

B

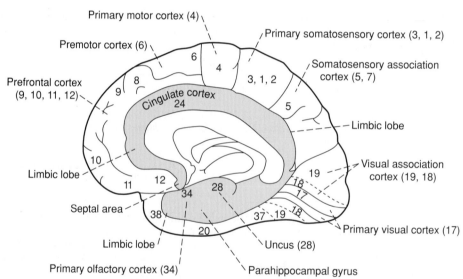

● **Figure 22-2** Some motor and sensory areas of the cerebral cortex. **(A)** Lateral convex surface of the hemisphere. **(B)** Medial surface of the hemisphere. The numbers refer to the Brodmann brain map (Brodmann's areas).

B. PARIETAL LOBE

1. In the **sensory cortex** (Brodmann's areas 3, 1, and 2), which is somatotopically organized (see Figure 22-2), destruction results in contralateral hemihypesthesia and astereognosis.

2. In the **superior parietal lobule** (Brodmann's areas 5 and 7), destruction results in contralateral astereognosis and sensory neglect.

3. In the **inferior parietal lobule** of the **dominant hemisphere**, damage results in Gerstmann's syndrome, which includes the following deficits:

   a. **Right and left confusion.**

   b. **Finger agnosia.**

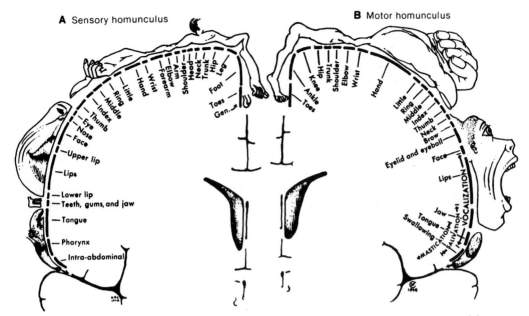

● **Figure 22-3** The sensory and motor homunculi. **(A)** Sensory representation in the postcentral gyrus. **(B)** Motor representation in the precentral gyrus. (Reprinted from W Penfield, T Rasmussen, *The cerebral cortex of man*. New York: Hafner, 1968:44, 57, with permission.)

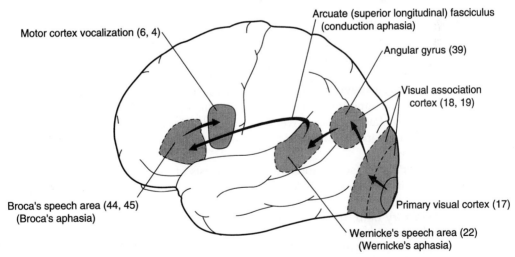

● **Figure 22-4** Cortical areas of the dominant hemisphere that play an important role in language production. The visual image of a word is projected from the visual cortex (Brodmann's area 17) to the visual association cortices (Brodmann's areas 18 and 19) and then to the angular gyrus (Brodmann's area 39). Further processing occurs in Wernicke's speech area (Brodmann's area 22), where the auditory form of the word is recalled. Through the arcuate fasciculus, this information reaches Broca's speech area (Brodmann's areas 44 and 45), where motor speech programs control the vocalization mechanisms of the precentral gyrus. Lesions of Broca's speech area, Wernicke's speech area, or the arcuate fasciculus result in dysphasia. (Reprinted from JD Fix, *BRS neuroanatomy*, 3rd ed. Baltimore: Lippincott Williams & Wilkins, 2003:377, with permission.)

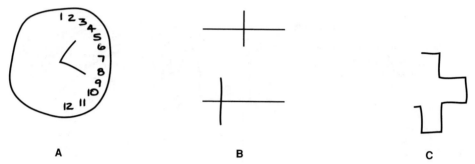

A   **B**   **C**

● **Figure 22-5** Testing for construction apraxia. **(A)** The patient was asked to copy the face of a clock. **(B)** The patient was asked to bisect a horizontal line. **(C)** The patient was asked to copy a cross. These drawings show contralateral neglect. The responsible lesion is found in the nondominant (right) parietal lobe. A left hemianopia, by itself, does not result in contralateral neglect.

       c. **Dysgraphia and dyslexia.**
       d. **Dyscalculia.**
       e. **Contralateral hemianopia or lower quadrantanopia.**
   4. In the **inferior parietal lobule of the nondominant hemisphere**, destruction results in the following deficits:
       a. **Topographic memory loss.**
       b. **Anosognosia.**
       c. **Construction apraxia** (Figure 22-5).
       d. **Dressing apraxia.**
       e. **Contralateral sensory neglect.**
       f. **Contralateral hemianopia or lower quadrantanopia.**

C. TEMPORAL LOBE
   1. In the **primary auditory cortex** (Brodmann's areas 41 and 42), unilateral destruction results in slight loss of hearing. Bilateral loss results in cortical deafness.
   2. **Wernicke's speech area** in the **dominant hemisphere** is found in the posterior part of the superior temporal gyrus (Brodmann's area 22). Destruction results in receptive, fluent aphasia (Wernicke's aphasia), in which the patient cannot understand any form of language. Speech is spontaneous, fluent, and rapid, but makes little sense.
   3. **Meyer's loop** (see Chapter 15 II.F.2) consists of the visual radiations that project to the inferior bank of the calcarine sulcus. Interruption causes contralateral upper quadrantanopia ("pie in the sky").
   4. **Olfactory bulb, tract,** and **primary cortex** (Brodmann's area 34) can see destruction that results in ipsilateral anosmia. An irritative lesion (psychomotor epilepsy) of the uncus results in olfactory and gustatory hallucinations.
       a. **Olfactory groove meningiomas** compress the olfactory tract and bulb, resulting in anosmia. See Foster Kennedy syndrome, Chapter 11.I.C.

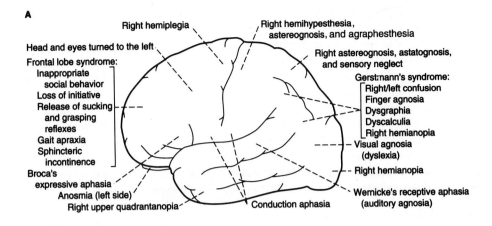

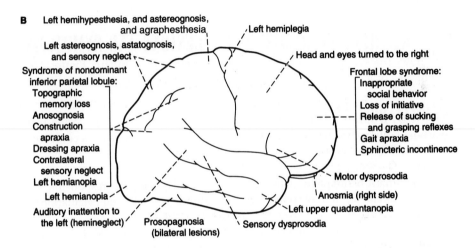

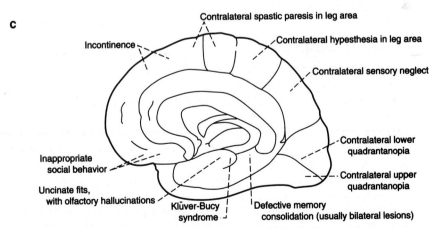

● **Figure 22-6** Focal destructive hemispheric lesions and the resulting symptoms. **(A)** Lateral convex surface of the dominant left hemisphere. **(B)** Lateral convex surface of the nondominant right hemisphere. **(C)** Medial surface of the nondominant hemisphere.

      b. **Esthesioneuroblastomas** (olfactory neuroblastomas) arise from bipolar sensory cells of the olfactory mucosa; they can extend through the cribriform plate into the anterior cranial fossa. Presenting symptoms are similar to those of the Foster Kennedy syndrome.

    5. In the **hippocampal cortex (archicortex)**, bilateral lesions result in the inability to consolidate short-term memory into long-term memory. Earlier memories are retrievable.

    6. In the **anterior temporal lobe**, including the **amygdaloid nucleus**, bilateral damage results in **Kläver-Bucy** syndrome, which consists of **psychic blindness** (visual agnosia), **hyperphagia**, docility, and **hypersexuality**.

    7. In the **inferomedial occipitotemporal cortex**, bilateral lesions result in the inability to recognize once-familiar faces (prosopagnosia).

  D. **OCCIPITAL LOBE.** Bilateral lesions cause cortical blindness. Unilateral lesions cause contralateral hemianopia or quadrantanopia.

IV. FOCAL DESTRUCTIVE HEMISPHERIC LESIONS AND SYMPTOMS

Figure 22-6A shows the symptoms of lesions in the dominant hemisphere. Figure 22-6B shows the symptoms of lesions in the nondominant hemisphere.

V. CEREBRAL DOMINANCE

This dominance is determined by the **Wada test.** Sodium amobarbital (Amytal) is injected into the carotid artery. If the patient becomes aphasic, the anesthetic was administered to the dominant hemisphere.

  A. The **dominant hemisphere** is usually the left hemisphere. It is responsible for **propositional language** (grammar, syntax, and semantics), speech, and calculation.

  B. The **nondominant hemisphere** is usually the right hemisphere. It is responsible for three-dimensional, or spatial, perception and nonverbal ideation. It also allows superior recognition of faces.

VI. SPLIT-BRAIN SYNDROME

(Figure 22-7). This syndrome is a disconnection syndrome that results from **transection** of the **corpus callosum.**

  A. The **dominant hemisphere** is better at vocal naming.

  B. The **nondominant, mute hemisphere** is better at pointing to a stimulus. A person cannot name objects that are presented to the nondominant visual cortex. A blindfolded person cannot name objects that are presented to the nondominant sensory cortex through touch.

  C. **TEST** (Figure 22-8). A subject views a composite picture of two half-faces (i.e., a chimeric, or hybrid, figure). The right side shows a man; the left side shows a woman. The picture is removed, and the subject is asked to describe what he saw. He may respond that he saw a man, but when asked to point to what he saw, he points to the woman.

  D. In a patient who has **alexia** in the left visual field, the verbal symbols seen in the right visual cortex have no access to the language centers of the left hemisphere.

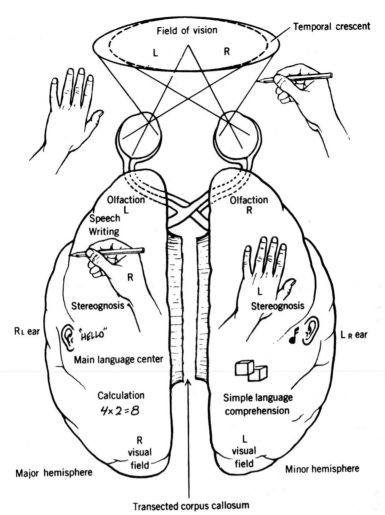

● **Figure 22-7** Functions of the split brain after transection of the corpus callosum. Tactile and visual perception is projected to the contralateral hemisphere, olfaction is perceived on the same side, and audition is perceived predominantly in the opposite hemisphere. The left (*L*) hemisphere is dominant for language. The right (*R*) hemisphere is dominant for spatial construction and nonverbal ideation. (Reprinted from CR Noback, RJ Demarest, *The human nervous system*. Malvern, PA: Lea & Febiger, 1991:416, with permission.)

VII OTHER LESIONS OF THE CORPUS CALLOSUM

A. ANTERIOR CORPUS CALLOSUM LESION may result in akinetic mutism or tactile anomia.

B. POSTERIOR CORPUS CALLOSUM (SPLENIUM) LESION may result in alexia without agraphia.

C. CALLOSOTOMY has been successfully used to treat "drop attacks" (colloid cyst of third ventricle).

VIII BRAIN AND SPINAL CORD TUMORS (see Chapter 1)

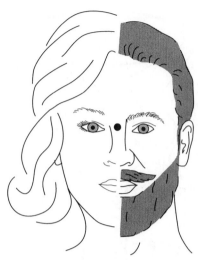

● **Figure 22-8** Chimeric (hybrid) figure of a face used to examine the hemispheric function of commissurotomized patients. The patient is instructed to fixate on the dot and is asked to describe what is seen. If the patient says that he or she sees the face of a man, the left hemisphere predominates in vocal tasks. If he or she is asked to point to the face and points to the woman, the right hemisphere predominates in pointing tasks.

Case Study

A 50-year-old woman was referred to neurology with a year-long history of poor memory and speech difficulties. She noted an inability to remember the names of common household objects and complained of forgetting her friends' names. She complained of becoming indecisive, such that she had significant difficulty in making straightforward decisions and in processing new information.

Physical Exam Findings

• On testing higher cortical function, her speech was somewhat rambling and hesitant, with word finding difficulty. The neurologic examination was otherwise normal.

Relevant Lab Findings

• Single-photon emission computed tomography cerebral perfusion disclosed markedly reduced perfusion in the left temporal and parietal lobes and the right posterior parietal regions.

Diagnosis

• Aphasia is a language disorder resulting from damage to brain regions responsible for language (left hemisphere). Onset may occur either suddenly, owing to trauma, or slowly, as in the case of a brain tumor. Aphasia impairs expression and understanding of language and reading and writing.

Chapter **23**

Neurotransmitters

 Key Concepts

1) In this chapter, the pathways of the major neurotransmitters are shown in separate brain maps.
2) Glutamate (GLU) is the major excitatory transmitter of the brain; GABA is the major inhibitory transmitter. Purkinje cells of the cerebellum are GABA-ergic.
3) In Alzheimer's disease, there is a loss of acetylcholinergic neurons in the basal nucleus of Meynert.
4) In Parkinson's disease, there is a loss of dopaminergic neurons in the substantia nigra.

I. IMPORTANT TRANSMITTERS AND THEIR PATHWAYS

A. **ACETYLCHOLINE** is the major transmitter of the peripheral nervous system, neuromuscular junction, parasympathetic nervous system, preganglionic sympathetic fibers, and postganglionic sympathetic fibers that innervate **sweat glands** and **some blood vessels** in the skeletal muscles (Figure 23-1). Acetylcholine is found in the neurons of the somatic and visceral motor nuclei in the brain stem and spinal cord. It is also found in the **basal nucleus of Meynert**, which degenerates in **Alzheimer's disease**.

B. **CATECHOLAMINES.** Figure 23-2 shows the biosynthetic pathway for catecholamines. Epinephrine, though a catecholamine, plays an insignificant role as a central nervous system neurotransmitter. In the body, epinephrine is found primarily in the adrenal medulla. In the central nervous system, it is restricted to small neuronal clusters in the brain stem (medulla).

    1. **Dopamine** (Figure 23-3) is depleted in patients with Parkinson's disease and increased in patients with schizophrenia. Dopamine is found in the arcuate nucleus of the hypothalamus. It is the **prolactin-inhibiting factor**. Its two major receptors are D_1 and D_2.

        a. **D_1 receptors** are postsynaptic. They activate adenylate cyclase and are excitatory.

        b. **D_2 receptors** are both postsynaptic and presynaptic. They inhibit adenylate cyclase and are inhibitory. Antipsychotic drugs block D_2 receptors.

    2. **Norepinephrine** (Figure 23-4) is the transmitter of most postganglionic sympathetic neurons. Antidepressant drugs enhance its transmission.

        a. Norepinephrine plays a role in **anxiety** states. **Panic attacks** are believed to result from paroxysmal discharges from the **locus ceruleus**, where norepinephrinergic neurons are found in the highest concentration. Most postsynaptic receptors of the locus ceruleus pathway are β_1 or β_2 receptors that activate adenylate cyclase and are excitatory.

Acetylcholine (ACh)

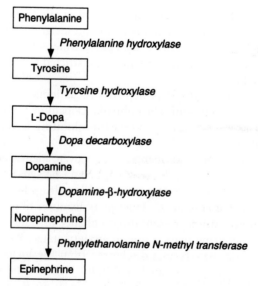

Neocortex

Local circuit neurons
in striatum (caudatoputamen)

Hippocampal formation

Nucleus basilis of Meynert in forebrain
(Alzheimer's disease)

Cranial nerve, motor neurons, and
preganglionic parasympathetic neurons

Spinal motor neurons
Autonomic preganglionic neurons

● **Figure 23-1** Distribution of acetylcholine-containing neurons and their axonal projections. The basal nucleus of Meynert projects to the entire cortex. This nucleus degenerates in patients with Alzheimer's disease. Striatal acetylcholine local circuit neurons degenerate in patients with Huntington's disease.

    b. The **catecholamine hypothesis of mood disorders** states that reduced norepinephrine activity is related to depression and that increased norepinephrine activity is related to mania.

C. **SEROTONIN [5-HYDROXYTRYPTAMINE (5-HT)]** is an indolamine (Figure 23-5). Serotonin-containing neurons are found only in the **raphe nuclei** of the brain stem.
    1. The **permissive serotonin hypothesis** states that when 5-HT activity is reduced, decreased levels of catecholamines cause depression and insomnia. In addition, when 5-HT activity is increased, elevated levels of catecholamines cause mania. Dysfunction of 5-HT may underlie obsessive-compulsive disorder.

Phenylalanine

Phenylalanine hydroxylase

Tyrosine

Tyrosine hydroxylase

L-Dopa

Dopa decarboxylase

Dopamine

Dopamine-β-hydroxylase

Norepinephrine

Phenylethanolamine N-methyl transferase

Epinephrine

● **Figure 23-2** Synthesis of catecholamines from phenylalanine. Epinephrine, which is derived from norepinephrine, is found primarily in the adrenal medulla.

Dopamine

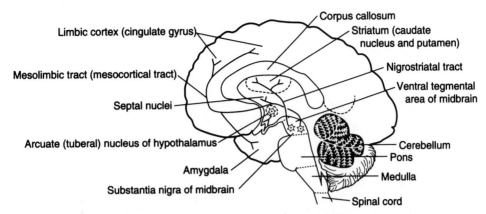

● **Figure 23-3** Distribution of dopamine-containing neurons and their projections. Two major ascending dopamine pathways arise in the midbrain: the nigrostriatal tract from the substantia nigra and the mesolimbic tract from the ventral tegmental area. In patients with Parkinson's disease, loss of dopaminergic neurons occurs in the substantia nigra and the ventral tegmental area. Dopaminergic neurons from the arcuate nucleus of the hypothalamus project to the portal vessels of the infundibulum. Dopaminergic neurons inhibit prolactin.

    2. Certain **antidepressants** increase 5-HT availability by reducing its reuptake. 5-HT agonists that bind $5\text{-}HT_{1A}$ and those that block $5\text{-}HT_2$ have antidepressant properties. Fluoxetine is a selective serotonin reuptake inhibitor.

D. OPIOID PEPTIDES (ENDOGENOUS OPIATES) induce responses similar to those of heroin and morphine.

    1. Endorphins include β-endorphin, which is the major endorphin found in the brain. It is one of the most powerful analgesics known (48 times more potent than morphine). Endorphins are found exclusively in the hypothalamus.

Norepinephrine (NE)

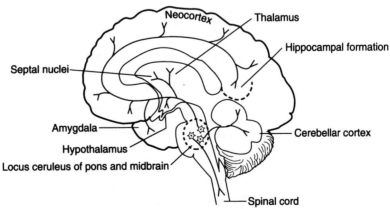

● **Figure 23-4** Distribution of norepinephrine-containing neurons and their projections. The locus ceruleus (located in the pons and midbrain) is the chief source of noradrenergic fibers. The locus ceruleus projects to all parts of the central nervous system.

Serotonin (5-HT)

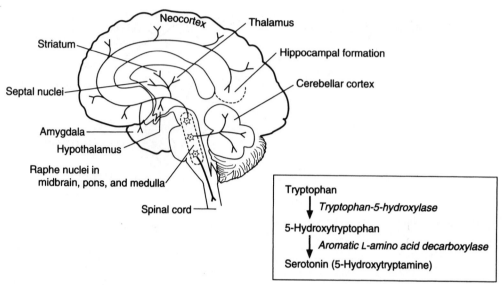

● **Figure 23-5** Distribution of 5-hydroxytryptamine (serotonin)-containing neurons and their projections. Serotonin-containing neurons are found in the nuclei of the raphe. They project widely to the forebrain, cerebellum, and spinal cord. The *inset* shows the synthetic pathway of serotonin.

2. **Enkephalins** are the most widely distributed and abundant opiate peptides. They are found in the highest concentration in the globus pallidus. Enkephalins coexist with dopamine, γ-aminobutyric acid (GABA), norepinephrine, and acetylcholine. They are colocalized in GABA-ergic pallidal neurons, and they play a role in pain suppression.

3. **Dynorphins** follow the distribution map for enkephalins.

E. NONOPIOID NEUROPEPTIDES

1. **Substance P** plays a role in **pain transmission**. It is most highly concentrated in the substantia nigra. It is also found in the dorsal root ganglion cells and substantia gelatinosa. It is colocalized with GABA in the striatonigral tract and plays a role in **movement disorders**. Substance P levels are **reduced** in patients with **Huntington's disease**.

2. **Somatostatin (somatotropin-release-inhibiting factor).** Somatostatinergic neurons from the anterior hypothalamus project their axons to the median eminence, where somatostatin enters the hypophyseal portal system and **regulates the release of growth hormone** and **thyroid-stimulating hormone**. The concentration of somatostatin in the neocortex and hippocampus is significantly **reduced** in patients with **Alzheimer's disease**. Striatal somatostatin levels are **increased** in patients with Huntington's disease.

F. AMINO ACID TRANSMITTERS

1. **Inhibitory amino acid transmitters**

   a. **GABA** (Figure 23-6) is the major inhibitory neurotransmitter of the brain. Purkinje, stellate, basket, and Golgi cells of the cerebellar cortex are GABA-ergic.

γ-Aminobutyric acid (GABA)

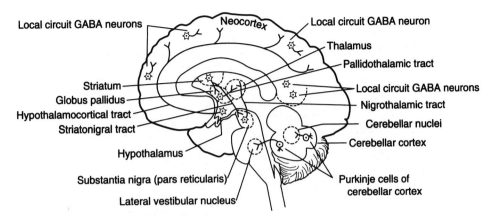

● **Figure 23-6** Distribution of γ-aminobutyric acid (*GABA*)-containing neurons and their projections. GABA-ergic neurons are the major inhibitory cells of the central nervous system. GABA local circuit neurons are found in the neocortex, hippocampal formation, and cerebellar cortex (Purkinje cells). Striatal GABA-ergic neurons project to the thalamus and subthalamic nucleus (not shown).

    (1) GABA-ergic striatal neurons project to the globulus pallidus and substantia nigra.

    (2) GABA-ergic pallidal neurons project to the thalamus.

    (3) GABA-ergic nigral neurons project to the thalamus.

    (4) GABA receptors (GABA-A and GABA-B) are intimately associated with benzodiazepine-binding sites. Benzodiazepines enhance GABA activity.

        (a) GABA-A receptors open chloride channels.

        (b) GABA-B receptors are found on the terminals of neurons that use another transmitter (i.e., norepinephrine, dopamine, serotonin). Activation of GABA-B receptors decreases the release of the other transmitter.

  b. **Glycine** is the major inhibitory neurotransmitter of the spinal cord. It is used by the Renshaw cells of the spinal cord.

2. **Excitatory amino acid transmitters**

  a. **Glutamate** (Figure 23-7). GLU is the **major excitatory transmitter of the brain.** Neocortical glutamatergic neurons project to the striatum, subthalamic nucleus, and thalamus.

    (1) GLU is the transmitter of the cerebellar granule cells.

    (2) GLU is also the transmitter of nonnociceptive, large, primary afferent fibers that enter the spinal cord and brain stem.

    (3) GLU is the transmitter of the corticobulbar and corticospinal tracts.

  b. **Aspartate.** A major excitatory transmitter of the brain, aspartate is the transmitter of the climbing fibers of the cerebellum. Neurons of climbing fibers are found in the inferior olivary nucleus.

  c. **Behavioral correlation.** GLU, through its N-methyl-D-aspartate (**NMDA**) **receptors,** plays a role in **long-term potentiation** (a memory process) of hippocampal neurons. GLU plays a role in **kindling** and subsequent **seizure activity.** Under certain conditions, glutamate and its analogs are **neurotoxic.**

  d. **Glutamate excitotoxicity.** GLU is released in the striatum and binds to its receptors on striatal neurons, resulting in an action potential. GLU is removed

Glutamate

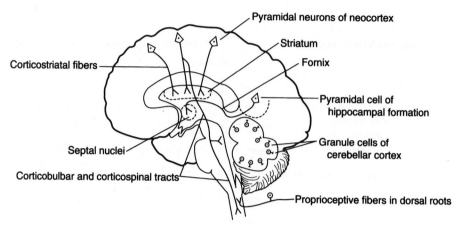

● Figure 23-7 Distribution of glutamate-containing neurons and their projections. Glutamate is the major excitatory transmitter of the central nervous system. Cortical glutamatergic neurons project to the striatum. Hippocampal and subicular glutamatergic neurons project through the fornix to the septal area and hypothalamus. The granule cells of the cerebellum are glutamatergic.

from the extracellular space by astrocytes. In Huntington's disease, GLU is bound to the NMDA receptor, resulting in an influx of calcium ions and subsequent cell death. This cascade of events with neuronal death most likely occurs in cerebrovascular accidents (stroke).

3. **Nitric oxide** is a recently discovered gaseous neurotransmitter that is produced when nitric oxide-synthase converts arginine to citrulline.

   a. It is located in the olfactory system, striatum, neocortex, hippocampal formation, supraoptic nucleus of the hypothalamus, and cerebellum.

   b. Nitric oxide is responsible for smooth-muscle relaxation of the corpus cavernosum and thus penile erection. It is also believed to play a role in memory formation because of its long-term potentiation in the hippocampal formation. In addition, nitric oxide functions as a nitrovasodilator in the cardiovascular system.

Ⅱ FUNCTIONAL AND CLINICAL CONSIDERATIONS

A. **PARKINSON'S DISEASE** results from degeneration of the dopaminergic neurons that are found in the pars compacta of the substantia nigra. It causes a reduction of dopamine in the striatum and substantia nigra (see Chapter 21, III.A).

B. **HUNTINGTON'S DISEASE (CHOREA)** results from a loss of acetylcholine- and GABA-containing neurons in the striatum (caudatoputamen). The effect is a loss of GABA in the striatum and substantia nigra (see Chapter 21, III.C).

C. **ALZHEIMER'S DISEASE** results from the degeneration of cortical neurons and cholinergic neurons in the **basal nucleus of Meynert**. It is associated with a 60% to 90% loss of choline acetyltransferase in the cerebral cortex. Histologically, **Alzheimer's disease is characterized by the presence of neurofibrillary tangles, senile (neuritic) plaques, amyloid substance, granulovacuolar degeneration, and Hirano bodies.**

D. **MYASTHENIA GRAVIS** results from autoantibodies against the nicotinic acetylcholine receptor on skeletal muscle. These antibodies block the postganglionic acetylcholine-binding site. Thymic cells augment B-cell production of autoantibodies. The cardinal manifestation is fatigable weakness of the skeletal muscle. The extraocular muscles, including the levator palpebrae, are usually involved. Edrophonium or neostigmine injection is used for diagnosis.

E. **LAMBERT-EATON MYASTHENIC SYNDROME** is caused by a presynaptic defect of acetylcholine release. It causes weakness in the limb muscles but not the bulbar muscles. Fifty percent of cases are associated with neoplasms (i.e., lung, breast, prostate). In these patients, muscle strength improves with use. In contrast, in patients with myasthenia gravis, muscle use results in muscle fatigue, and autonomic dysfunction includes dry mouth, constipation, impotence, and urinary incontinence.

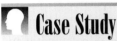 # Case Study

A 60-year-old man presents with progressive stiffness accompanied by difficulty in walking and going down stairs. He has an expressionless face and a vacant, staring gaze. Examination revealed limited ocular motility in all directions. What is the most likely symptomatic therapy?

Relevant Physical Exam Findings

- Tremor at rest, with pill-rolling motion of the hand
- Rigidity observed when the patient's relaxed wrist is flexed and extended
- Bradykinesia

Diagnosis

- Parkinson's disease is a progressive neurodegenerative disorder associated with a loss of dopaminergic nigrostriatal neurons. Often, patients are given levodopa combined with carbidopa. Nerve cells use levodopa to make dopamine to compensate for the loss of nigrostriatal neurons, whereas carbidopa delays the conversion of levodopa into dopamine until it reaches the brain.

Chapter 24

Apraxia, Aphasia, and Dysprosody

 Key Concepts

1) Be able to differentiate Broca's aphasia from Wernicke's aphasia.
2) What is conduction aphasia?

APRAXIA is the inability to perform motor activities in the presence of intact motor and sensory systems and normal comprehension.

A. IDEOMOTOR APRAXIA (IDIOKENETIC APRAXIA)
1. The disorder results in loss of the ability to perform intransitive or imaginary gestures; the inability to perform complicated motor tasks (e.g., saluting, blowing a kiss, or making the "V" for victory sign)
2. The lesion is in Wernicke's area.
3. **Bucco-facial or facial-oral apraxia** is a type of idiomotor apraxia; facial apraxia is the most common type of apraxia.

B. IDEATIONAL APRAXIA (IDEATORY APRAXIA)
1. The inability to demonstrate the use of real objects (e.g., ask the patient to smoke a pipe, a multistep complex sequence)
2. A misuse of objects owing to a disturbance of identification (agnosia)
3. The lesion in Wernicke's area

C. CONSTRUCTION APRAXIA, the inability to draw or construct a geometric figure (e.g., the face of a clock). If the patient draws only the right half of the clock, this condition is called *hemineglect*, and the lesion is located in the right inferior parietal lobule.

D. GAIT APRAXIA, the inability to use the lower limbs properly. The patient has difficulty in lifting his feet from the floor, a frontal lobe sign seen with **normal-pressure hydrocephalus (gait apraxia, dementia, incontinence).**

APHASIA is impaired or absent communication by speech, writing, or signs (i.e., loss of the capacity for spoken language). The lesions are located in the dominant hemisphere. Associate the following symptoms and lesion sites with the appropriate aphasia (Figure 24-1).

A. BROCA'S (MOTOR) APHASIA
1. Lesion in frontal lobe, in the inferior frontal gyrus (Brodmann's areas 44 and 45)
2. Good comprehension

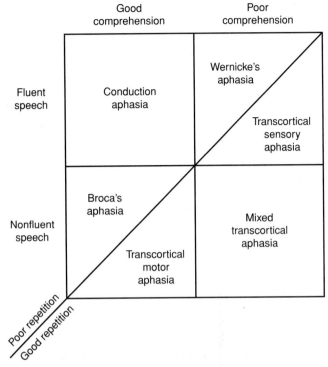

● **Figure 24-1** The "aphasia square" makes it easy to differentiate the six most common "national board" aphasias. Broca's, conduction and Wernicke's aphasias are all characterized by poor repetition. (Adapted from J Miller, N Fountain, *Neurology recall.* Baltimore: Williams & Wilkins, 1997:35, with permission.)

    3. Effortful speech
    4. Dysarthric speech
    5. Telegraphic speech
    6. Nonfluent speech
    7. Poor repetition
    8. Contralateral lower facial and upper limb weakness

B. WERNICKE'S (SENSORY) APHASIA
    1. Lesion in posterior temporal lobe, in the superior temporal gyrus (Brodmann's area 22)
    2. Poor comprehension
    3. Fluent speech
    4. Poor repetition
    5. Quadrantanopia
    6. Paraphasic errors
        a. **Non sequiturs** (Latin, "does not follow"): statements irrelevant to the question asked
        b. **Neologisms:** words with no meaning
        c. **Driveling speech**

C. CONDUCTION APHASIA
    1. **Transection of the arcuate fasciculus;** the arcuate fasciculus interconnects Brodmann's speech area with Wernicke's speech area.
    2. Poor repetition

   3. Good comprehension
   4. Fluent speech

D. TRANSCORTICAL MOTOR APHASIA
   1. Poor comprehension
   2. Good repetition
   3. Nonfluent speech

E. TRANSCORTICAL MIXED APHASIA
   1. Poor comprehension
   2. Good repetition
   3. Nonfluent speech

F. TRANSCORTICAL SENSORY APHASIA
   1. Poor comprehension
   2. Good repetition
   3. Fluent speech

G. GLOBAL APHASIA. Resulting from a lesion of the perisylvian area, which contains Broca's and Wernicke's areas, global aphasia combines all of the symptoms of Broca's and Wernicke's aphasias.

H. THALAMIC APHASIA. A dominant thalamic syndrome, thalamic aphasia closely resembles a thought disorder of patients with schizophrenia and chronic drug-induced psychosis. Symptoms include fluent paraphasic speech with normal comprehension and repetition.

I. BASAL GANGLIA. Diseases of the basal ganglia may cause aphasia. Lesions of the anterior basal ganglia result in nonfluent aphasia. Lesions of the posterior basal ganglia result in fluent aphasia.

J. WATERSHED INFARCTS. Such infarcts are areas of infarction in the boundary zones of the anterior, middle, and posterior cerebral arteries. These areas are vulnerable to hypoperfusion and thus may separate Broca's and Wernicke's speech areas from the surrounding cortex. These infarcts cause the motor, mixed, and sensory transcortical aphasias.

III DYSPROSODY is a nondominant hemispheric language deficit that serves propositional language. Emotionality, inflection, melody, emphasis, and gesturing are affected.

A. EXPRESSIVE DYSPROSODY results from a lesion that corresponds to Broca's area but is located in the nondominant hemisphere. Patients cannot express emotion or inflection in their speech.

B. RECEPTIVE DYSPROSODY results from a lesion that corresponds to Wernicke's area but is located in the nondominant hemisphere. Patients cannot comprehend the emotionality or inflection in the speech they hear.

Case Study

A 7-year-old boy presents with difficulty in articulating words, though he can hear words and understand their meaning. His mother noted he had difficulty in breast-feeding during infancy.

Relevant Physical Exam Findings

- Limited ability to produce speech sounds
- Groping for correct placement of the tongue, lips, and jaw during speech
- Omission of words in sentences
- Atypical facial expressions

Diagnosis

- Apraxia results when sounds do not easily form into words. A complex coordination of lips, tongue, and throat muscles is required to articulate words.

Appendix I

Table of Cranial Nerves

Cranial Nerve	Type	Origin	Function	Course
I–Olfactory	SVA	Bipolar olfactory (olfactory epithelium in roof of nasal cavity)	Smell (olfaction)	Central axons project to the olfactory bulb via the cribriform plate of the ethmoid bone.
II–Optic	SSA	Retinal ganglion cells	Vision	Central axons converge at the optic disk and form the optic nerve, which enters the skull via the optic canal. Optic nerve axons terminate in the lateral geniculate bodies.
III–Oculomotor				
Parasympathetic	GVE	Edinger-Westphal nucleus (rostral midbrain)	Sphincter muscle of iris; ciliary muscle	Axons exit the midbrain in the interpeduncular fossa, traverse the cavernous sinus, and enter the orbit via the superior orbital fissure.
Motor	GSE	Oculomotor nucleus (rostral midbrain)	Superior, inferior, and medial recti muscles; inferior oblique muscle; levator palpebrae muscle	
IV–Trochlear	GSE	Trochlear nucleus (caudal midbrain)	Superior oblique muscle	Axons decussate in superior medullary velum, exit dorsally inferior to the inferior colliculi, encircle the midbrain, traverse the cavernous sinus, and enter the orbit via the superior orbital fissure.
V–Trigeminal				
Motor	SVE	Motor nucleus CN V (midpons)	Muscles of mastication and tensor tympani muscle	Ophthalmic nerve exits via the superior orbital fissure; maxillary nerve exits via the foramen rotundum; mandibular nerve exits via the foramen ovale; ophthalmic and maxillary nerves traverse the cavernous sinus; GSA fibers enter the spinal trigeminal tract of CN V.
Sensory	GSA	Trigeminal ganglion and mesencephalic nucleus CN V (rostral pons and midbrain)	Tactile, pain, and thermal sensation from the face; the oral and nasal cavities; and the supratentorial dura	

Cranial Nerve	Type	Origin	Function	Course
VI–Abducent	GSE	Abducent nucleus (caudal pons)	Lateral rectus muscle	Axons exit the pons from the inferior pontine sulcus, traverse the cavernous sinus, and enter the orbit via the superior orbital fissure.
VII–Facial				
Parasympathetic	GVE	Superior salivatory nucleus (caudal pons)	Lacrimal gland (via sphenopalatine ganglion); sub-mandibular and sublingual glands (via submandibular ganglion)	Axons exit the pons in the cere-bellar pontine angle and enter the internal auditory meatus; motor fibers traverse the facial canal of the temporal bone and exit via the stylomastoid fora-men; taste fibers traverse the chorda tympani and lingual nerve; GSA fibers enter the spinal trigeminal tract of CN V; SVA fibers enter the tract.
Motor	SVE	Facial nucleus (caudal pons)	Muscles of facial expression; stapedius muscle	
Sensory	GSA	Geniculate ganglion (temporal bone)	Tactile sensation to skin of ear	
Sensory	SVA	Geniculate ganglion	Taste sensation from the anterior two-thirds of tongue (via chorda tympani)	
VIII–Vestibulocochlear				
Vestibular nerve	SSA	Vestibular ganglion (internal auditory meatus)	Equilibrium (inner-vates hair cells of semicircular ducts, saccule, and utricle)	Vestibular and cochlear nerves join in the internal auditory meatus and enter the brain stem in the cerebellopontine angle; vestibular nerve projects to the vestibular nuclei and the flocculonodular lobe of the cerebellum; cochlear nerve pro-jects to the cochlear nuclei.
Cochlear nerve		Spinal ganglion (modiolus of temporal bone)	Hearing (innervates hair cells of the organ of Corti)	
IX–Glossopharyngeal				
Parasympathetic	GVE	Inferior salivatory nucleus (rostral medulla)	Parotid gland (via the otic ganglion)	Axons exit (motor) and enter (sensory) medulla from the postolivary sulcus; axons exit and enter the skull via jugular foramen; GSA fibers enter the spinal trigeminal tract of CN V; GVA and SVA fibers enter the solitary tract.
Motor	SVE	Nucleus ambiguous (rostral medulla)	Stylopharyngeus muscle	
Sensory	GSA	Superior ganglion (jugular foramen)	Tactile sensation to external ear	
Sensory	GVA	Inferior (petrosal) ganglion (in jugular foramen)	Tactile sensation to posterior third of tongue, pharynx, middle ear, and auditory tube, input from carotid sinus and carotid body	
Sensory	SVA	Inferior (petrosal) ganglion (in jugular foramen)	Taste from posterior third of the tongue	

(continued)

Cranial Nerve	Type	Origin	Function	Course
X–Vagal				
Parasympathetic	GVE	Dorsal nucleus of CN X (medulla)	Viscera of the thoracic and abdominal cavities to the left colic flexure [via terminal (mural) ganglia]	Axons exit (motor) and enter (sensory) medulla from the postolivary sulcus; axons exit and enter the skull via the jugular foramen; GSA fibers enter the spinal trigeminal tract of CN V; GVA and SVA fibers enter the solitary tract.
Motor	SVE	Nucleus ambiguus (midmedulla)	Muscles of the larynx and pharynx	
Sensory	GSA	Superior ganglion (jugular foramen)	Tactile sensation to the external ear	
Sensory	GVA	Inferior (nodose) ganglion (in jugular foramen)	Mucous membranes of the pharynx, larynx, esophagus, trachea, and thoracic and abdominal viscera to the left colic flexure	
Sensory	SVA	Inferior (nodose) ganglion (in jugular foramen)	Taste from the epiglottis	
XI–Accessory				
Motor (cranial)		Nucleus ambiguus (medulla)	Intrinsic muscles of the larynx (except the cricothyroid muscle) via recurrent laryngeal nerve	Axons from the cranial division exit the medulla from the postolivary sulcus and join the vagal nerve; axons from spinal division exit the spinal cord, ascend through the foramen magnum, and exit the skull via the jugular foramen.
Motor (spinal)		Ventral horn neurons C1–C6	Sternocleidomastoid and trapezius muscles	
XII–Hypoglossal		Hypoglossal nucleus (medulla)	Intrinsic and extrinsic muscles of the tongue (except the palatoglossus muscle)	Axons exit from the preolivary sulcus of the medulla and exit the skull via the hypoglossal canal.

SVA, special visceral afferent; SSA, special somatic afferent; GVE, general visceral efferent; GSE, general somatic efferent; SVE, special visceral efferent; GSA, general somatic afferent; GVA, general visceral afferent; CN, cranial nerve.

Table of Common Neurological Disease States

Disease State	Characteristics
Acoustic neuroma	Derived from the Schwann cell sheath investing cranial nerve VIII; accounts for most tumors located in the cerebellopontine angle
Agnosia	Disorder of skilled movement; not due to paresis
Alzheimer's disease	Most common cause of dementia; anatomical pathology shows neurofibrillary tangles and senile plaques microscopically; cortical atrophy of the temporal lobe
Anencephaly	Neural tube defect in which the cerebrum and cerebellum are malformed while the hindbrain is intact
Aneurysm (cerebral)	Pathological localized dilatation in the wall of an artery
Anosmia	Inability to detect odors; may result from congenital defects (Kallman syndrome) or trauma
Anosognosia	Translates to "denial of illness" because patients denied their hemiplegia early after stroke
Anton syndrome	Form of cortical blindness in which the patient denies the visual impairment; results from damage to primary visual and visual association cortex of the occipital lobe
Aphasia	Language disorder resulting from stroke, trauma, or tumor of the left cerebral hemisphere; affects the patient's ability to produce and comprehend speech as well as the ability to hear and read words
Apraxia	Disorder of skilled movement in which the patient is not paralyzed but cannot perform basic activities; involves inferior parietal lobe and premotor cortex
Argyll-Robertson pupil	Small, irregular pupil that functions normally in accommodation but cannot react to light; often associated with neurosyphilis
Arnold-Chiari malformation	Congenital malformation of the hindbrain involving inferior displacement of the medulla, fourth ventricle, and cerebellum through foramen magnum
Astereognosis	Inability to recognize a familiar object when placed in the hand of a patient with eyes closed
Balint's syndrome	Characterized by poor visuomotor coordination and inability to understand visual objects; results from stroke of posterior cerebral artery
Benedikt's syndrome	Oculomotor palsy on the side of the lesion in the ventral midbrain (fascicular segment of cranial nerve III)
Cauda equina syndrome	Lower motor neuron lesion characterized by pain of the lower back and lower limb as well as bladder and bowel dysfunction; results from lesion of nerve roots of cauda equina

(continued)

Disease State	Characteristics
Chorea	Literally means "to dance;" patients cannot maintain a sustained posture; demonstrate "milkmaid's grip" and "harlequin's tongue"
Chromatolysis	Disintegration of Nissl substance in a neuronal cell body following damage to the cells' axon
Conus medullaris syndrome	Characterized by both upper and lower motor neuron signs, including back and leg pain, paresthesias and weakness, perineal or saddle anesthesia, and urorectal dysfunction; often results from acute disc herniation
Dandy-Walker malformation	Congenital malformation characterized by underdevelopment of the cerebellar vermis, dilation of the fourth ventricle, and enlargement of the posterior cranial fossa; developmental delays, enlarged head circumference, and symptoms of hydrocephalus may be observed
Duret's hemorrhage	Small punctate hemorrhages of the midbrain and pons resulting from arteriole stretching during the primary injury; may also result during transtentorial herniation as a secondary injury
Dysgraphia	Learning disability characterized by difficulty in expressing thoughts in writing; associated with extremely poor handwriting; results from head trauma
Dyskinesia	Involuntary movements often associated with extrapyramidal disorders such as Parkinson's disease
Dyslexia	Impairment in the ability to translate written visual images into meaningful language; common learning disability in children
Dysmetria	Lack of coordinated of movements of upper limb and eyes; characterized by under- or overshooting the intended position; closely related condition to intention tremor; may be associated with multiple sclerosis, in which it results from cerebellar lesions
Dysprosody	Characterized by alterations in rhythm and intonation of spoken words (prosody); associated with apraxia of speech; results from left frontal lesions adjacent to the Broca's area
Dystaxia	Literally means "no order"; involves loss of ability to grossly control skeletal muscles; characterized by dysphagia, dysarthria, and stiffness of movement
Foster Kennedy syndrome	Combination of papilledema in one eye and optic nerve atrophy in the other; characterized by visual loss in the atrophic eye; may also result from more distal remote ischemia or demyelination
Gerstmann's syndrome	Characterized by four signs, including writing disability (agraphia; dysgraphia), failure to understand arithmetic (acalculia; dyscalculia), inability to distinguish right from left, and an inability to identify fingers (finger agnosia)
Guillain-Barré syndrome	Peripheral neuropathy characterized by weakness affecting the lower extremities first, progressing superiorly to the arms and facial muscles; any sensory loss presents as loss of proprioception and areflexia
Hemianesthesia	Unilateral loss of sensation from the face; loss of pain and temperature sense on the contralateral side of the body
Hemianopia	Loss of half of the visual field
Hemiballism	Involuntary movements of the extremities, trunk, and mandible; associated with diseases of the basal nuclei (ganglia)
Hemiparesis	Unilatearl partial paralysis, resulting from lesions of the corticospinal tract
Herniation	High intracranial pressure shifts of the brain and brain stem relative to the falx cerebri, the tentorium cerebelli, and through foramen magnum
Hirschsprung's disease	Congenital disorder involving blockage of the colon due to dysfunction of smooth muscle contraction; results from abnormal neural crest cell migration into the myenteric plexus during embryonic development
Holoprosencephaly	Failure of the prosencephalon (forebrain) to develop

Disease State	Characteristics
Horner's syndrome	Interruption of sympathetic innervation to the eye; characterized by three primary signs, including ptosis, miosis, and anhidrosis
Jugular foramen syndrome	Trauma to or tumor at the jugular foramen, with resultant paralysis of cranial nerves IX, X, and IX; often results from a basilar skull fracture
Kluver-Bucy syndrome	Lesion of medial temporal lobes and amygdala; characterized by oral and tactile exploratory behavior (inappropriate licking or touching in public); hypersexuality; flattened emotions (placidity)
Lambert-Eaton syndrome	Disorder of presynaptic neuromuscular transmission; impaired release of acetylcholine, resulting in proximal muscle weakness and abnormal tendon reflexes
Lateral medullary syndrome	Also known as Wallenberg's syndrome and posterior inferior cerebellar artery (PICA) syndrome; involves difficulty in swallowing and speaking; results from occlusion of PICA resulting in infarction of the lateral part of the medulla
Locked-in syndrome	Complete paralysis of all voluntary muscles of the body except the extraocular muscles; patients fully alert but cannot move; only movements of the eyes and blinking are possible; results from stroke in the pons
Lou Gehrig's disease [amyotrophic lateral sclerosis (ALS)]	Progressive degeneration of upper and lower motor neurons, resulting in hyperreflexia and spasticity (degeneration of the lateral corticospinal tracts) as well as weakness, atrophy, and fasciculations (due to muscle denervation)
Meningomyelocele	Cyst containing brain tissue, cerebrospinal fluid, and the meninges, protruding through a congenital defect in the skull; results from failure of the neural tube to close during gestation
Multiple sclerosis	Autoimmune disorder in which antibodies are created against proteins in the myelin sheath; results in inflammation of myelin and the nerves that it invests; causes scarring (sclerosis), which slows or blocks neurotransmission
Myasthenia gravis	Literally means "grave muscle"; chronic autoimmune neuromuscular disease characterized by weakness of the skeletal muscles of the body that worsens during periods of activity and improves after rest
Nystagmus	Involuntary rhythmic shaking or wobbling of the eyes; results from a pathological process that damages one or more components of the vestibular system, including the semicircular canals, otolithic organs, and vestibulocerebellum
Parinaud's syndrome	Bacterial infection of the eye, related to pinkeye, or conjunctivitis; tularemia may infect the eye by direct or indirect entry of the bacteria into the eye
Parkinson's disease	Disorder of the basal nuclei (ganglia) that results in resting tremor of a limb, slowness of movement (bradykinesia), rigidity of the limbs or trunk, and postural instability
Raynaud's disease	Vascular disease reducing blood flow to the extremities when exposed to environmental stimuli, including temperature changes or stress
Romberg sign	Results of a neurologic exam used to assess the dorsal columns of the spinal cord involved in proprioception; a positive Romberg sign indicates sensory ataxia, whereas a negative Romberg sign suggests cerebellar ataxia
Subclavian steal syndrome	Occlusion of subclavian artery proximal to the origin of the vertebral artery; involves reversed blood flow in the vertebral artery; so named because it was thought that blood was stolen by the ipsilateral vertebral artery from the contralateral vertebral artery
	Cyst (syrinx) forms and expands within the spinal cord, destroying central

(continued)

Disease State	Characteristics
Syringomelia	tissue in the cord; results in pain, weakness, and stiffness in the trunk and limbs
Tabes dorsalis	Slow degeneration of the neurons in the dorsal columns of the spinal cord; results in abnormal proprioceptive signals
Tic douloureux	Also known as trigeminal neuralgia; unilateral, severe, stabbing pain of the face, particularly jaw, cheek, or lip
Wallerian degeneration	Process of degeneration of the axons distal to a site of transection
Watershed infarct	Occurs at the junction of two nonanastomosing arterial systems; often between branches of the anterior and middle cerebral arteries
Wilson's disease	Also known as hepatolenticular degeneration; genetic disorder in which copper accumulates in the liver and basal nuclei (ganglia), specifically in the putamen and globus pallidus (lenticular nucleus)
Weber's syndrome	Also known as superior alternating hemiplegia; involves oculomotor nerve palsy and contralateral hemiparesis or hemiplegia; results from midbrain infarction as a result of occlusion of the posterior cerebral artery
Wernicke-Korsakoff syndrome	Neurologic disorder resulting from thiamine deficiency; usually caused by malnutrition, common in alcoholic patients; may present with vision changes, loss of muscle coordination, memory loss

Glossary

abasia Inability to walk.

abulia Inability to perform voluntary actions or to make decisions; seen in bilateral frontal lobe disease.

accommodation Increase in thickness of the lens needed to focus a near external object on the retina.

adenohypophysis Anterior lobe of the pituitary gland, derived from Rathke's pouch.

adenoma sebaceum Cutaneous lesion seen in tuberous sclerosis.

Adie pupil (Myotonic pupil) A tonic pupil, usually large, that constricts very slowly to light and convergence; generally unilateral and frequently occurs in young women with absent knee or ankle reflexes.

afferent pupil (Marcus Gunn pupil) A pupil that reacts sluggishly to direct light stimulation; caused by a lesion of the afferent pathway (e.g., multiple sclerosis involving the optic nerve).

agenesis Failure of a structure to develop (e.g., agenesis of the corpus callosum).

ageusia Loss of the sensation of taste (gustation).

agnosia Lack of the sensory-perceptional ability to recognize objects; visual, auditory, and tactile.

agraphesthesia Inability to recognize figures "written" on the skin.

agraphia Inability to write; seen in Gerstmann's syndrome.

akathisia (acathisia) Inability to remain in a sitting position; motor restlessness; may appear after the withdrawal of neuroleptic drugs.

akinesia Absence or loss of the power of voluntary motion; seen in Parkinson's disease.

akinetic mutism State in which patient can move and speak but cannot be prompted to do so; due to bilateral occlusion of the anterior cerebral artery or midbrain lesions.

alar plate Division of the mantle zone that gives rise to sensory neurons; receives sensory input from the dorsal root ganglia.

albuminocytologic dissociation Elevated cerebrospinal fluid (CSF) protein with a normal CSF cell count; seen in Guillain-Barré syndrome.

alexia Visual aphasia; word or text blindness; loss of the ability to grasp the meaning of written or printed words; seen in Gerstmann's syndrome.

Alzheimer's disease Condition characterized pathologically by the presence of senile plaques, neurofibrillary tangles, granulovacuolar degeneration, Hirano bodies, and amyloid deposition; patients are demented with severe memory loss.

alternating hemianesthesia Ipsilateral facial anesthesia and a contralateral body anesthesia; results from a pontine or medullary lesion involving the spinal trigeminal tract and the spinothalamic tract.

alternating hemiparesis Ipsilateral cranial nerve palsy and a contralateral hemiparesis (e.g., alternating abducent hemiparesis).

altitudinal hemianopia Defect in which the upper or lower half of the visual field is lost.

amaurosis fugax Transient monocular blindness usually related to carotid artery stenosis or, less often, to embolism of retinal arterioles.

amnesia Disturbance or loss of memory; seen with bilateral medial temporal lobe lesions.

amusia Form of aphasia characterized by the loss of ability to express or recognize simple musical tones.

amyotrophic lateral sclerosis (ALS) A nonhereditary motor neuron disease affecting both upper and lower motor neurons; characterized by muscle weakness, fasciculations, fibrillations, and giant motor units on electromyography. There are no sensory deficits in ALS. It is also called *Lou Gehrig's disease.*

amyotrophy Muscle wasting or atrophy.

analgesia Insensibility to painful stimuli.

anencephaly Failure of the cerebral and cerebellar hemispheres to develop; results from failure of the anterior neuropore to close.

anesthesia State characterized by the loss of sensation.

aneurysm Circumscribed dilation of an artery (e.g., berry aneurysm).

anhidrosis Absence of sweating; found in Horner syndrome.

anisocoria Pupils that are unequal in size; found in a third-nerve palsy and Horner's syndrome.

anomia Anomic aphasia; the inability to name objects; may result from a lesion of the angular gyrus.

anosmia Olfactory anesthesia; loss of the sense of smell.

anosognosia Ignorance of the presence of disease.

Anton syndrome (visual anosognosia) Lack of awareness of being cortically blind; bilateral occipital lesions affecting the visual association cortex.

aphasia Impaired or absent communication by speech, writing, or signs; loss of the capacity for spoken language.

aphonia Loss of the voice.

apparent enophthalmos Ptosis seen in Horner's syndrome that makes the eye appear as if it is sunk back into the orbit.

apraxia Disorder of voluntary movement; the inability to execute purposeful movements; the inability to properly use an object (e.g., a tool.)

aprosodia (aprosody) Absence of normal pitch, rhythm, and the variation of stress in speech.

area postrema Chemoreceptor zone in the medulla that responds to circulating emetic substances; it has no blood–brain barrier.

areflexia Absence of reflexes.

Argyll Robertson pupil Pupil that responds to convergence but not to light (near light dissociation); seen in neurosyphilis and lesions of the pineal region.

Arnold-Chiari malformation Characterized by herniation of the caudal cerebellar vermis and cerebellar tonsils through the foramen magnum; associated with lumbar myelomeningocele, dysgenesis of the corpus callosum, and obstructive hydrocephalus.

arrhinencephaly Characterized by agenesis of the olfactory bulbs; results from malformation of the forebrain; associated with trisomy 13–15 and holoprosencephaly.

ash-leaf spots Hypopigmented patches typically seen in tuberous sclerosis.

astasia-abasia Inability to stand or walk.

astatognosia Position agnosia; the inability to recognize the position or disposition of an extremity or digit in space.

astereognosis (stereoanesthesia) Tactile amnesia; the inability to judge the form of an object by touch.

asterixis Flapping tremor of the outstretched arms seen in hepatic encephalopathy and Wilson's disease.

ataxia (incoordination) Inability to coordinate muscles during the execution of voluntary movement (e.g., cerebellar and posterior column ataxia).

athetosis Slow, writhing, involuntary, purposeless movements seen in Huntington's disease (chorea).

atresia Absence of a normal opening(s) (e.g., atresia of the outlet foramina of the fourth ventricle, which results in Dandy-Walker syndrome).

atrophy Muscle wasting; seen in lower motor neuron (LMN) disease.

auditory agnosia Inability to interpret the significance of sound; seen in Wernicke's dysphasia/aphasia.

autotopagnosia (somatotopagnosia) Inability to recognize parts of the body; seen with parietal lobe lesions.

Babinski sign Extension of the great toe in response to plantar stimulation (S-I); indicates corticospinal (pyramidal) tract involvement.

Balint syndrome (optic ataxia) Condition characterized by a failure to direct oculomotor function in the exploration of space; failure to follow a moving object in all quadrants of the field once the eyes are fixed on the object.

ballism Dyskinesia resulting from damage to the subthalamic nucleus; consists in violent flailing and flinging of the contralateral extremities.

basal plate Division of the mantle zone that gives rise to lower motor neurons (LMNs).

Bell's palsy Idiopathic facial nerve paralysis.

Benedikt's syndrome Condition characterized by a lesion of the midbrain affecting the intraaxial oculomotor fibers, medial lemniscus, and cerebellothalamic fibers.

berry aneurysm Small, saccular dilation of a cerebral artery; ruptured berry aneurysms are the most common cause of nontraumatic subarachnoid hemorrhage.

blepharospasm Involuntary recurrent spasm of both eyelids; effective treatment is injections of botulinum toxin into the orbicularis oculi muscles.

blood–brain barrier Tight junctions (zonulae occludentes) of the capillary endothelial cells.

blood–cerebrospinal fluid (CSF) barrier Tight junctions (zonulae occludentes) of the choroid plexus.

bradykinesia Extreme slowness in movement; seen in Parkinson's disease.

Broca's aphasia Difficulty in articulating or speaking language; found in the dominant inferior frontal gyrus; also called *expressive, anterior, motor,* or *nonfluent aphasia.*

bulbar palsy Progressive bulbar palsy; a lower motor neuron (LMN) paralysis affecting primarily the motor nuclei of the medulla; the prototypic disease is amyotrophic lateral sclerosis (ALS), characterized by dysphagia, dysarthria, and dysphonia.

caloric nystagmus Nystagmus induced by irrigating the external auditory meatus with either cold or warm water; remember COWS mnemonic: cold, opposite, warm, same.

cauda equina Sensory and motor nerve rootlets found below the vertebral level L-2; lesions of the cauda equina result in motor and sensory defects of the leg.

cerebral edema Abnormal accumulation of fluid in the brain; associated with volumetric enlargement of brain tissue and ventricles; may be vasogenic, cytotoxic, or both.

cerebral palsy Defect of motor power and coordination resulting from brain damage; the most common cause is hypoxia and asphyxia manifested during parturition.

Charcot-Bouchard aneurysm Miliary aneurysm; microaneurysm; rupture of this type of aneurysm is the most common cause of intraparenchymal hemorrhage; most commonly found in the basal ganglia.

Charcot-Marie-Tooth disease Most commonly inherited neuropathy affecting lower motor neurons (LMNs) and dorsal root ganglion cells; also called *peroneal muscular atrophy.*

cherry-red spot (macula) Seen in Tay-Sachs disease; resembles a normal-looking retina; the retinal ganglion cells surrounding the fovea are packed with lysosomes and no longer appear red.

chorea Irregular, spasmodic, purposeless, involuntary movements of the limbs and facial muscles; seen in Huntington's disease.

choreiform Resembling chorea.

choreoathetosis Abnormal body movements of combined choreic and athetoid patterns.

chromatolysis Disintegration of Nissl substance following transection of an axon (axotomy).

clasp-knife spasticity Resistance that is felt initially and then fades like the opening of a pocketknife when a joint is moved briskly; seen with corticospinal lesions.

clonus Contractions and relaxations of a muscle (e.g., ankle or wrist clonus); seen with corticospinal tract lesions.

cog-wheel rigidity Rigidity characteristic of Parkinson's disease. Bending a limb results in ratchetlike movements.

conduction aphasia Aphasia in which patient has relatively normal comprehension and spontaneous speech but difficulty with repetition; results from a lesion of the arcuate fasciculus, which interconnects the Broca and Wernicke areas.

confabulation Making bizarre and incorrect responses; seen in Wernicke-Korsakoff psychosis.

construction apraxia Inability to draw or construct geometric figures; frequently seen in nondominant parietal lobe lesions.

conus medullaris syndrome Condition characterized by paralytic bladder, fecal incontinence, impotence, and perianogenital sensory loss; involves segments S3–Co.

Corti organ (spiral organ) Structure containing hair cells responding to sounds that induce vibrations of the basilar membrane.

COWS (mnemonic) Cold, opposite, warm, same; cold water injected into the external auditory meatus results in nystagmus to the opposite side; warm water injected into the external auditory meatus results in nystagmus to the ipsilateral or same side.

Creutzfeldt-Jakob disease Rapidly progressing dementia, supposedly caused by an infectious prion; histologic picture is that of a spongiform encephalopathy; classic triad is dementia, myoclonic jerks, and typical electroencephalographic (EEG) findings; similar spongiform encephalopathies are scrapie (in sheep), kuru, as well as Gerstmann-Sträussler-Scheinker disease, which is characterized by cerebellar ataxia and dementia.

crocodile tears syndrome Lacrimation during eating; results from a facial nerve injury proximal to the geniculate ganglion; regenerating preganglionic salivatory fibers are misdirected to the pterygopalatine ganglion, which projects to the lacrimal gland.

cupulolithiasis Dislocation of the otoliths of the utricular macula that causes benign positional vertigo.

cycloplegia Paralysis of accommodation (CN III) (i.e., paralysis of the ciliary muscle).

Dandy-Walker malformation Characterized by congenital atresia of the foramina of Luschka and Magendie, hydrocephalus, posterior fossa cyst, and dilatation of the fourth ventricle; associated with agenesis of the corpus callosum.

decerebrate posture (rigidity) Posture in comatose patients in which the arms are overextended, the legs are extended, the hands are flexed, and the head is extended. The causal lesion is in the rostral midbrain.

decorticate posture (rigidity) Posture in comatose patients in which the arms are flexed and the legs are extended. The causal lesion (anoxia) involves both hemispheres.

dementia pugilistica (punch-drunk syndrome) Condition characterized by dysarthria, parkinsonism, and dementia. Ventricular enlargement and fenestration of the septum pellucidum are common; most common cause of death is subdural hematoma.

diabetes insipidus Condition characterized by excretion of large amounts of pale urine; results from inadequate output of the antidiuretic hormone (ADH) from the hypothalamus.

diplegia Paralysis of the corresponding parts on both sides of the body.

diplopia Double vision.

doll's eyes maneuver (oculocephalic reflex) Moving the head of a comatose patient with intact brainstem; results in a deviation of the eyes to the opposite direction.

Down syndrome Condition that results from a chromosomal abnormality (trisomy 21). Alzheimer's disease is common in Down syndrome after the age of 40 years.

dressing apraxia Loss of the ability to dress oneself; frequently seen in nondominant parietal lobe lesions.

Duret's hemorrhages Midbrain and pontine hemorrhages due to transtentorial (uncal) herniation.

dysarthria Disturbance of articulation (e.g., vagal nerve paralysis).

dyscalculia Difficulty in performing calculations; seen in lesions of the dominant parietal lobule.

dysdiadochokinesia Inability to perform rapid, alternating movements (e.g., supination and pronation); seen in cerebellar disease.

dysesthesia Impairment of sensation; disagreeable sensation produced by normal stimulation.

dyskinesias Movement disorders attributed to pathologic states of the striatal (extrapyramidal) system. Movements are generally characterized as insuppressible, stereotyped, and automatic.

dysmetria Past pointing; a form of dystaxia seen in cerebellar disease.

dysnomia Dysnomic (nominal) aphasia; difficulty in naming objects or persons; seen with some degree in all aphasias.

dysphagia Difficulty in swallowing; dysaglutition.

dysphonia Difficulty in speaking; hoarseness.

dyspnea Difficulty in breathing.

dysprosodia (dysprosody) Difficulty of speech in producing or understanding the normal pitch, rhythm, and variation in stress. Lesions are found in the nondominant hemisphere.

dyssynergia Incoordination of motor acts; seen in cerebellar disease.

dystaxia Difficulty in coordinating voluntary muscle activity; seen in posterior column and cerebellar disease.

dystonia (torsion dystonia) Sustained involuntary contractions of agonists and antagonists (e.g., torticollis); may be caused by the use of neuroleptics.

dystrophy When applied to muscle disease, it implies abnormal development and genetic determination.

edrophonium (Tensilon) Diagnostic test for myasthenia gravis.

embolus Plug formed by a detached thrombus.

emetic Agent that causes vomiting; see area postrema.

encephalocele Result of herniation of meninges and brain tissue through an osseous defect in the cranial vault.

encephalopathy Any disease of the brain.

enophthalmos Recession of the globe (eyeball) with the orbit.

epicritic sensation Discriminative sensation; posterior column–medial lemniscus modalities.

epilepsy Chronic disorder characterized by paroxysmal brain dysfunction caused by excessive neuronal discharge (seizure); usually associated with some alteration of consciousness; may be associated with a reduction of γ-aminobutyric acid (GABA).

epiloia Tuberous sclerosis, a neurocutaneous disorder; characterized by dementia, seizures, and adenoma sebaceum.

epiphora Tear flow due to lower eyelid palsy (CN VII).

exencephaly Congenital condition in which the skull is defective with the brain exposed; seen in anencephaly.

extrapyramidal (motor) system Motor system including the striatum (caudate nucleus and putamen), globus pallidus, subthalamic nucleus, and substantia nigra; also called the *striatal (motor) system*.

facial apraxia Inability to perform facial movements on command.

fasciculations Visible twitching of muscle fibers seen in lower motor neuron (LMN) disease.

festination Acceleration of a shuffling gait seen in Parkinson's disease.

fibrillations Nonvisible contractions of muscle fibers found in lower motor neuron (LMN) disease.

flaccid paralysis Complete loss of muscle power or tone resulting from lower motor neuron (LMN) disease.

folic acid deficiency Common cause of megaloblastic anemia; may also cause fetal neural tube defects (e.g., spina bifida).

gait apraxia Diminished capacity to walk or stand; frequently seen with bilateral frontal lobe disease.

gegenhalten Paratonia; a special type of resistance to passive stretching of muscles; seen with frontal lobe disease.

Gerstmann's syndrome Condition characterized by right-left confusion, finger agnosia, dysgraphia, and dyscalculia; results from a lesion of the dominant inferior parietal lobule.

glioma Tumor (neoplasm) derived from glial cells.

global aphasia Difficulty with comprehension, repetition, and speech.

graphesthesia Ability to recognize figures "written" on the skin.

hallucination False sensory perception with localizing value.

hematoma Localized mass of extravasated blood; a contained hemorrhage (e.g., subdural or epidural).

hemianhidrosis Absence of sweating on half of the body or face; seen in Horner's syndrome.

hemianopia Hemianopsia; loss of vision in one-half of the visual field of one or both eyes.

hemiballism Dyskinesia resulting from damage to the subthalamic nucleus; consists of violent flinging and flailing movements of the contralateral extremities.

hemiparesis Slight paralysis affecting one side of the body; seen in stroke involving the internal capsule.

hemiplegia Paralysis of one side of the body.

herniation Pressure-induced protrusion of brain tissue into an adjacent compartment; may be transtentorial (uncal), subfalcine (subfalcial), or transforaminal (tonsillar).

herpes simplex encephalitis Disorder characterized by headache, behavioral changes (memory), and seizures; the most common cause of encephalitis in the central nervous system. The temporal lobes are preferentially the target of hemorrhagic necrosis.

heteronymous Referring to noncorresponding halves or quadrants of the visual fields (e.g., binasal hemianopia).

hidrosis Sweating, perspiration, and diaphoresis.

Hirano bodies Eosinophilic, rodlike structures (inclusions) found in the hippocampus in Alzheimer's disease.

holoprosencephaly Failure of the prosencephalon to diverticulate and form two hemispheres.

homonymous Referring to corresponding halves or quadrants of the visual fields (e.g., left homonymous hemianopia).

Horner's syndrome Oculosympathetic paralysis consisting of miosis, hemianhidrosis, mild ptosis, and apparent enophthalmos.

hydranencephaly Condition in which the cerebral cortex and white matter are replaced by membranous sacs; believed to be the result of circulatory disease.

hydrocephalus Condition marked by excessive accumulation of cerebrospinal fluid (CSF) and dilated ventricles.

hygroma Collection of cerebrospinal fluid (CSF) in the subdural space.

hypacusis Hearing impairment.

hypalgesia Decreased sensibility to pain.

hyperacusis Abnormal acuteness of hearing; the result of a facial nerve paralysis (e.g., Bell's palsy).

hyperphagia Gluttony; overeating, as seen in hypothalamic lesions.

hyperpyrexia High fever, as seen in hypothalamic lesions.

hyperreflexia An exaggeration of muscle stretch reflexes (MSRs) as seen with upper motor neuron lesions (UMNs); a sign of spasticity.

hyperthermia Increased body temperature; seen with hypothalamic lesions.

hypertonia Increased muscle tone; seen with upper motor neuron (UMN) lesions.

hypesthesia (hypoesthesia) Diminished sensitivity to stimulation.

hypokinesia Diminished or slow movement; seen in Parkinson's disease.

hypophysis Pituitary gland.

hypothermia Reduced body temperature; seen in hypothalamic lesions.

hypotonia Reduced muscle tone; seen in cerebellar disease.

ideational or sensory apraxia Characterized by the inability to formulate the ideational plan for executing the several components of a complex multistep act (e.g., patient cannot go through the steps of lighting a cigarette when asked to); occurs most frequently in diffuse cerebral degenerating disease (e.g., Alzheimer's disease, multiinfarct dementia).

ideomotor or "classic" apraxia (ideokinetic apraxia) Inability to button one's clothes when asked; inability to comb one's hair when asked; inability to manipulate tools (e.g., hammer or screwdriver), although patient can explain their use; and inability to pantomime actions on request.

idiopathic Denoting a condition of an unknown cause (e.g., idiopathic Parkinson's disease).

infarction Sudden insufficiency of blood supply caused by vascular occlusion (e.g., emboli or thrombi), resulting in tissue necrosis (death).

intention tremor Tremor that occurs when a voluntary movement is made; a cerebellar tremor.

internal ophthalmoplegia Paralysis of the iris and ciliary body caused by a lesion of the oculomotor nerve.

internuclear ophthalmoplegia (INO) Medial rectus palsy on attempted conjugate lateral gaze caused by a lesion of the medial longitudinal fasciculus (MLF).

intraaxial Refers to structures found within the neuraxis; within the brain or spinal cord.

ischemia Local anemia caused by mechanical obstruction of the blood supply.

junction scotoma Results from a lesion of decussating fibers from the inferior nasal retinal quadrant that loop into the posterior part of the contralateral optic nerve; in the contralateral upper temporal quadrant.

Kayser-Fleischer ring Visible deposition of copper in Descemet's membrane of the corneoscleral margin; seen in Wilson's disease (hepatolenticular degeneration).

Kernig's sign Test method: subject lies on back with thigh flexed to a right angle, then tries to extend the leg. This movement is impossible with meningitis.

kinesthesia Sensory perception of movement, muscle sense; mediated by the posterior column–medial lemniscus system.

Klüver-Bucy syndrome Characterized by psychic blindness, hyperphagia, and hypersexuality; results from bilateral temporal lobe ablation including the amygdaloid nuclei.

labyrinthine hydrops Excess of endolymphatic fluid in the membranous labyrinth; cause of Ménière's disease.

lacunae Small infarcts associated with hypertensive vascular disease.

Lambert-Eaton myasthenic syndrome Condition that results from a defect in presynaptic acetylcholine (ACh) release; 50% of patients have a malignancy (e.g., lung or breast tumor).

lead-pipe rigidity Rigidity characteristic of Parkinson's disease.

Lewy bodies Eosinophilic, intracytoplasmic inclusions found in the neurons of the substantia nigra in Parkinson's disease.

Lhermitte's sign Electriclike shocks extending down the spine caused by flexing the head; due to damage of the posterior columns.

lipofuscin (ceroid) Normal inclusion of many neurons and glial cells; increases as the brain ages.

Lish nodules Pigmented hamartomas of the iris seen in neurofibromatosis type 1.

lissencephaly (agyria) Results from failure of the germinal matrix neuroblasts to reach the cortical mantle and form the gyri. The surface of the brain remains smooth.

"locked-in" syndrome Results from infarction of the base of the pons. Infarcted structures include the corticobulbar and corticospinal tracts, leading to quadriplegia and paralysis of the lower cranial nerves; patients can communicate only by blinking or moving their eyes vertically.

locus ceruleus Pigmented (neuromelanin) nucleus found in the pons and midbrain; contains the largest collection of norepinephrinergic neurons in the brain.

macrographia (megalographia) Large handwriting, seen in cerebellar disease.

magnetic gait Patient walks as if feet were stuck to the floor; seen in normal-pressure hydrocephalus (NPH).

medial longitudinal fasciculus (MLF) Fiber bundle found in the dorsomedial tegmentum of the brain stem just under the fourth ventricle; carries vestibular and ocular motor axons, which mediate vestibuloocular reflexes (e.g., nystagmus). Severance of this tract results in internuclear ophthalmoplegia (INO).

Mees lines Transverse lines on fingernails and toenails; due to arsenic poisoning.

megalencephaly Large brain weighing more than 1800 g.

meningocele Protrusion of the meninges of the brain or spinal cord through an osseous defect in the skull or vertebral canal.

meningoencephalocele Protrusion of the meninges and the brain through a defect in the occipital bone.

meroanencephaly Less severe form of anencephaly in which the brain is present in rudimentary form.

microencephaly (micrencephaly) A small brain weighing less than 900 g. The adult brain weighs approximately 1400 g.

micrographia Small handwriting, seen in Parkinson's disease.

microgyria (polymicrogyria) Small gyri; cortical lamination pattern not normal; seen in the Arnold-Chiari syndrome.

Millard-Gubler syndrome Alternating abducent and facial hemiparesis; an ipsilateral sixth and seventh nerve palsy and a contralateral hemiparesis.

mimetic muscles Muscles of facial expression; innervated by facial nerve (CN VII).

miosis Constriction of the pupil; seen in Horner's syndrome.

Möbius syndrome Congenital oculofacial palsy; consists of a congenital facial diplegia (CN VII) and a convergent strabismus (CN VI).

mononeuritis multiplex Vasculitic inflammation of several different nerves (e.g., polyarteritis nodosa).

MPTP (1-methyl-4-phenyl-1,3,3,6-tetrahydropyridine) **poisoning** Results in the destruction of the dopaminergic neurons in the substantia nigra, thus resulting in parkinsonism.

multiinfarct dementia Dementia due to the cumulative effect of repetitive infarcts; strokes characterized by cortical sensory, pyramidal, and bulbar and cerebellar signs, which result in permanent damage; primarily seen in hypertensive patients.

multiple sclerosis Classic myelinoclastic disease in which the myelin sheath is destroyed, with the axon remaining intact; characterized by exacerbations and remissions, with paresthesias, double vision, ataxia, and incontinence; cerebrospinal fluid (CSF) findings include increased gamma globulin, increased beta globulin, presence of oligoclonal bands, and increased myelin basic protein.

muscular dystrophy X-linked myopathy characterized by progressive weakness, fiber necrosis, and loss of muscle cells; two most common types are Duchenne's and myotonic muscular dystrophy.

mydriasis Dilation of the pupil; seen in oculomotor paralysis.

myelopathy Disease of the spinal cord.

myeloschisis Cleft spinal cord resulting from failure of the neural folds to close or from failure of the posterior neuropore to close.

myoclonus Clonic spasm or twitching of a muscle or group of muscles, as seen in juvenile myoclonic epilepsy; composed of single jerks.

myopathy Disease of the muscle.

myotatic reflex Monosynaptic muscle stretch reflex (MSR).

neglect syndrome Results from a unilateral parietal lobe lesion; neglect of one-half of the body and of extracorporeal space; simultaneous stimulation results in extinction of one of the stimuli; loss of optokinetic nystagmus on one side.

Negri bodies Intracytoplasmic inclusions observed in rabies; commonly found in the hippocampus and cerebellum.

neuraxis Unpaired part of the central nervous system (CNS): spinal cord, rhombencephalon, and diencephalon.

neurilemma (neurolemma) Sheath of Schwann. Schwann cells (neurilemmal cells) produce the myelin sheath in the peripheral nervous system (PNS).

neurofibrillary tangles Abnormal double helical structures found in the neurons of Alzheimer's patients.

neurofibromatosis (von Recklinghausen disease) A neurocutaneous disorder. Neurofibromatosis type 1 consists predominantly of peripheral lesions (e.g., café au lait spots, neurofibromas, Lish nodules, schwannomas), whereas type 2 consists primarily of intracranial lesions (e.g., bilateral acoustic schwannomas and gliomas).

neurohypophysis Posterior lobe of the pituitary gland; derived from the downward extension of the hypothalamus, the infundibulum.

neuropathy Disorder of the nervous system.

Nissl bodies/substance Rough endoplasmic reticulum found in the nerve cell body and dendrites but not in the axon.

nociceptive Capable of appreciation or transmission of pain.

normal-pressure hydrocephalus Characterized by normal cerebrospinal fluid (CSF) pressure and the clinical triad dementia, gait dystaxia (magnetic gait), and urinary incontinence. Shunting is effective; mnemonic is wacky, wobbly, wet.

nucleus basalis of Meynert Contains the largest collection of cholinergic neurons in the brain; located in the forebrain between the anterior perforated substance and the globus pallidus; neurons degenerate in Alzheimer's disease.

nystagmus To-and-fro oscillations of the eyeballs; named after the fast component; seen in vestibular and cerebellar disease.

obex Caudal apex of the rhomboid fossa; marks the beginning of the "open medulla."

Ondine curse Inability of patient to breathe while sleeping; results from damage to the respiratory centers of the medulla.

optokinetic nystagmus Nystagmus induced by looking at moving stimuli (targets); also called *railroad nystagmus*.

otitis media Infection of the middle ear, which may cause conduction deafness; may also cause Horner's syndrome.

otorrhea Discharge of cerebrospinal fluid (CSF) via the ear canal.

otosclerosis New bone formation in the middle ear resulting in fixation of the stapes; the most frequent cause of progressive conduction deafness.

palsy Paralysis; often used to connote partial paralysis or paresis.

papilledema Choked disk; edema of the optic disk; caused by increased intracranial pressure (e.g., tumor, epi- or subdural hematoma).

paracusis Impaired hearing; an auditory illusion or hallucination.

paralysis Loss of muscle power due to denervation; results from a lower motor neuron (LMN) lesion.

paraphrasia Paraphasia; a form of aphasia in which a person substitutes one word for another, resulting in unintelligible speech.

paraplegia Paralysis of both lower extremities.

paresis Partial or incomplete paralysis.

paresthesia Abnormal sensation such as tingling, pricking, or numbness; seen with posterior column disease (e.g., tabes dorsalis).

Parinaud's syndrome Lesion of the midbrain tegmentum resulting from pressure of a germinoma, a tumor of the pineal region. The patient has a paralysis of upward gaze.

Pick's disease Dementia affecting primarily the frontal lobes; always spares the posterior one-third of the superior temporal gyrus; clinically indistinguishable from Alzheimer's disease.

pill-rolling tremor Tremor at rest; seen in Parkinson's disease.

planum temporale Auditory association cortex found posterior to the transverse gyri of Heschl on the inferior bank of the lateral sulcus; a part of Wernicke's area; larger on the left side in males.

poikilothermia Inability to thermoregulate; seen with lesions of the posterior hypothalamus.

polydipsia Frequent drinking; seen in lesions of the hypothalamus (diabetes insipidus).

polyuria Frequent micturition; seen with hypothalamic lesions (diabetes insipidus).

porencephaly Cerebral cavitation caused by localized agenesis of the cortical mantle; the cyst is lined with ependyma.

presbycusis (presbyacusia) Inability to perceive or discriminate sounds as part of the aging process; due to atrophy of the organ of Corti.

progressive supranuclear palsy Characterized by supranuclear ophthalmoplegia, primarily a downgaze paresis followed by paresis of other eye movements. As the disease progresses, the remainder of the motor cranial nerves becomes involved.

proprioception Reception of stimuli originating from muscles, tendons, and other internal tissues. Conscious proprioception is mediated by the dorsal column–medial lemniscus system.

prosopagnosia Difficulty in recognizing familiar faces.

protopathic sensation Pain, temperature, and light (crude) touch sensation; the modalities mediated by the spinothalamic tracts.

pseudobulbar palsy (pseudobulbar supranuclear palsy) Upper motor neuron (UMN) syndrome resulting from bilateral lesions that interrupt the corticobulbar tracts. Symptoms include difficulties with articulation, mastication, and deglutition; results from repeated bilateral vascular lesions.

psychic blindness Type of visual agnosia seen in the Klüver-Bucy syndrome.

psychosis Severe mental thought disorder.

ptosis Drooping of the upper eyelid; seen in Horner's syndrome and oculomotor nerve paralysis (CN III).

pyramidal (motor) system Voluntary motor system consisting of upper motor neurons (UMNs) in the corticobulbar and corticospinal tracts.

quadrantanopia Loss of vision in one quadrant of the visual field in one or both eyes.

quadriplegia Tetraplegia; paralysis of all four limbs.

rachischisis Spondyloschisis; failure of the vertebral arches to develop and fuse and form the neural tube.

raphe nuclei Paramedian nuclei of the brain stem that contain serotoninergic (5-hydroxytryptamine) neurons.

Rathke's pouch Ectodermal outpocketing of the stomodeum; gives rise to the adenohypophysis (anterior lobe of the pituitary gland).

retrobulbar neuritis Optic neuritis frequently caused by the demyelinating disease multiple sclerosis.

rhinorrhea Leakage of cerebrospinal fluid (CSF) via the nose.

rigidity Increased muscle tone in both extensors and flexors; seen in Parkinson's disease; cog-wheel rigidity and lead-pipe rigidity.

Romberg's sign On standing with feet together and closing eyes, subject loses balance; a sign of dorsal column ataxia.

saccadic movement Quick jump of the eyes from one fixation point to another. Impaired saccades are seen in Huntington's disease.

scanning speech (scanning dysarthria) Breaking up of words into syllables; typical of cerebellar disease and multiple sclerosis (e.g., I DID not GIVE any TOYS TO my son FOR CHRISTmas).

schizophrenia Psychosis characterized by a disorder in the thinking processes (e.g., delusions and hallucinations); associated with dopaminergic hyperactivity.

scotoma Blind spot in the visual field.

senile (neuritic) plaques Swollen dendrites and axons, neurofibrillary tangles, and a core of amyloid; found in Alzheimer's disease.

shagreen spots Cutaneous lesions found in tuberous sclerosis.

shaken baby syndrome Three major physical findings: retinal hemorrhages, large head circumference, and bulging fontanelle. Eighty percent of the subdural hemorrhages are bilateral.

sialorrhea (ptyalism) Excess of saliva (e.g., drooling), seen in Parkinson's disease.

simultanagnosia Inability to understand the meaning of an entire picture even though some parts may be recognized; the inability to perceive more than one stimulus at a time.

singultus Hiccups; frequently seen in the posterior inferior cerebellar artery (PICA) syndrome.

somatesthesia (somesthesia) Bodily sensations that include touch, pain, and temperature.

spasticity Increased muscle tone (hypertonia) and hyperreflexia [exaggerated muscle stretch reflexes (MSRs)]; seen in upper motor neuron (UMN) lesions.

spastic paresis Partial paralysis with hyperreflexia resulting from transection of the corticospinal tract.

spina bifida Neural tube defect with variants: spina bifida occulta, spina bifida with meningocele, spina bifida with meningomyelocele, and rachischisis; results from failure of the vertebral laminae to close in the midline.

status marmoratus Hypermyelination in the putamen and thalamus; results from perinatal asphyxia; clinically presents as double athetosis.

stereoanesthesia (astereognosis) Inability to judge the form of an object by touch.

"stiff-man syndrome" A myopathy characterized by progressive and permanent stiffness of the muscles of the back and neck and spreading to involve the proximal muscles of the extremities. The syndrome is caused by a disturbance of the inhibitory action of Renshaw cells in the spinal cord.

strabismus Lack of parallelism of the visual axes of the eyes; squint; heterotropia.

striae medullares (of the rhombencephalon) Fiber bundles that divide the rhomboid fossa into a rostral pontine part and a caudal medullary half.

stria medullaris (of the thalamus) Fiber bundle extending from the septal area to the habenular nuclei.

stria terminalis Semicircular fiber bundle extending from the amygdala to the hypothalamus and septal area.

Sturge-Weber syndrome Neurocutaneous congenital disorder including a port-wine stain (venous angioma) and calcified leptomeningeal angiomatoses (railroad track images seen on plain film); seizures occur in up to 90% of patients.

subclavian steal syndrome Occlusion of the subclavian artery, proximal to the vertebral artery, resulting in a shunting of blood down the vertebral and into the ipsilateral subclavian artery. Physical activity of the ipsilateral arm may cause signs of vertebrobasilar insufficiency (dizziness or vertigo).

sulcus limitans Groove separating the sensory alar plate from the motor basal plate; extends from the spinal cord to the mesencephalon.

sunset sign Downward look by eyes, in which the sclerae are above the irides and the upper eyelids are retracted; seen in congenital hydrocephalus and in progressive supranuclear palsy.

swinging flashlight sign Test to diagnose a relevant afferent pupil. Light shone into the afferent pupil results in a small change in pupil size bilaterally, and light shone into the normal pupil results in a decrease in pupil size in both eyes.

sympathetic apraxia Motor apraxia in the left hand; seen in lesions of the dominant frontal lobe.

syringomyelia Cavitation of the cervical spinal cord results in bilateral loss of pain and temperature sensation and wasting of the intrinsic muscles of the hands. Syringes may be found in the medulla (syringobulbia) and pons (syringopontia) and in Arnold-Chiari malformation.

tabes dorsalis Locomotor ataxia; progressive demyelination and sclerosis of the dorsal columns and roots; seen in neurosyphilis.

tactile agnosia Inability to recognize objects by touch.

tardive dyskinesia Syndrome of repetitive, choreoathetoid movements frequently affecting the face; results from treatment with antipsychotic agents.

Tay-Sachs disease (GM_2 gangliosidosis) Best-known inherited metabolic disease of the central nervous system (CNS); characterized by motor seizures, dementia, and blindness; a cherry-red spot (macula) occurs in 90% of cases; caused by a deficiency of hexosaminidase A; affects Ashkenazi Jews.

tethered cord syndrome (filum terminale syndrome) Characterized by numbness of the legs and feet, foot drop, loss of bladder control, and impotence.

thrombus Clot in an artery that is formed from blood constituents; gives rise to an embolus.

tic douloureux Trigeminal neuralgia.

tinnitus Ringing in the ear(s); seen with irritative lesions of the cochlear nerve (e.g., acoustic neuroma).

titubation A head tremor in the anteroposterior direction, often accompanying midline cerebellar lesions; also a staggering gait.

tremor Involuntary, rhythmic, oscillatory movement.

tuberous sclerosis (Bourneville's disease) Neurocutaneous disorder characterized by the trilogy of mental retardation, seizures, and adenoma sebaceum. Cutaneous lesions include periungual fibromas, shagreen patches, and ash-leaf spots.

uncinate fit Form of psychomotor epilepsy, including hallucinations of smell and taste; results from lesions of the parahippocampal gyrus (uncus).

upper motor neurons (UMNs) Cortical neurons that give rise to the corticospinal and corticobulbar tracts. Destruction of UMNs or their axons results in a spastic paresis. Some authorities include brain stem neurons that synapse on lower motor neurons (LMNs) (i.e., neurons from the red nucleus).

vertigo Sensation of whirling motion due to vestibular disease.

visual agnosia Inability to recognize objects by sight.

von Hippel-Lindau disease Disorder characterized by lesions of the retina and cerebellum; retinal and cerebellar hemangioblastomas. Non–central nervous system (CNS) lesions may include renal, epididymal, and pancreatic cysts, as well as renal carcinoma.

Wallenberg's syndrome Condition characterized by hoarseness, cerebellar ataxia, anesthesia of the ipsilateral face and contralateral body, and cranial nerve signs of dysarthria, dysphagia, dysphonia, vertigo, and nystagmus; results from infarction of the lateral medulla due to occlusion of the vertebral artery or its major branch, the posterior inferior cerebellar artery (PICA); Horner's syndrome is frequently found on the ipsilateral side.

Wallerian degeneration Anterograde degeneration of an axon and its myelin sheath after axonal transection.

Weber's syndrome Lesion of the midbrain basis pedunculi involving the root fibers of the oculomotor nerve and the corticobulbar and cortospinal tracts.

Werdnig-Hoffman syndrome (spinal muscular atrophy) Early childhood disease of the anterior horn cells [lower motor neuron (LMN) disease].

Wernicke's aphasia Difficulty in comprehending spoken language; also called *receptive, posterior, sensory,* or *fluent aphasia.*

witzelsucht Inappropriate facetiousness and silly joking; seen with frontal lobe lesions.

Index

Page numbers followed by "*f*" indicate figure; those followed by "*t*" indicate table.